Healing Springs

HEALING SPRINGS

A HISTORY OF THE SPRINGS
AND THE SURROUNDING AREA

Raymond P. Boylston

SANDLAPPER PUBLISHING CO., INC.
ORANGEBURG, SOUTH CAROLINA 29115

Published by Sandlapper Publishing Co., Inc.
Orangeburg, South Carolina 29115

Cover photograph © Larry Price
Larry Price Photography, 1783 Ashleigh Road, Williston, S.C. 29853
Telephone (803)259-7366

Cover design by Raymond P. Boylston

Manufactured in the United States of America

Library of Congress Cataloging-in-Publication Data

Boylston, Ray, 1930–
    Healing Springs : a history of the springs and the surrounding area /
Raymond P. Boylston.— 1st ed.
        p. cm.
    Includes bibliographical references.
    ISBN 0-87844-175-1 (trade pbk. : alk. paper)
1. Healing Springs Region (S.C.)—History.   I. Title.
    F279.H325B69 2004
    975.7'79—dc22

                                                    2004010754

DEDICATION

This book is dedicated to my wife, Bobbie Weeks Boylston, for her support and extensive assistance. Without her transcribing my scribbled notes and her many long hours on the computer, this book would never have been completed.

ACKNOWLEDGEMENTS

Many people have made significant contributions to this book—among them, Samuel L. Boylston, H. Flowe Trexler, Dan I. Ross, Jimmie Page Gunter, Bill Odom, Rev. David Grubbs of Healing Springs Baptist Church, Hemrick Salley, Jr., and Stanley McDonald. Myrtle Quattlebaum of Healing Springs provided extensive information and valuable assistance in reviewing the book. A special thanks to the many contributors to the *Barnwell County Heritage* book published in 1994 for their descriptions of life around Healing Springs and Blackville. I thank H. Flowe Trexler for allowing me to use much of the book material. I would also like to thank the Blackville Area Historical Society for information provided. Extensive research was conducted at the Barnwell County Library, South Carolina Department of Archives and History, South Caroliniana Library, Orangeburg County Historical Society Archives, Richland County Library, North Carolina Office of Archives and History, and the Blackville Library. This book would not have been written without the assistance and cooperation of these individuals and groups.

TABLE OF CONTENTS

Healing Springs

PREFACE

In the 1930s my aunt, Ruby Boylston, from Spring-field, South Carolina, took me on my first visit to Healing Springs, a few miles south of South Edisto River on Highway 3, the Springfield-to-Blackville road. She told me the water had healing powers and we should stop at the springs and drink the clear, cool water each time we drove to Blackville.

For the past sixty years I have continued this tradition. The springs have always been important to me. I learned at an early age that my ancestors settled a few miles north of Healing Springs along the south bank of South Edisto River in the late 1700s. Their farm, Oak Grove, was located near Boylston Landing. As my brother Sam and I dug deeper into our family history, we learned more and more about Healing Springs, the town of Blackville, and Barnwell County. It became obvious the springs were an important and interesting part of South Carolina history. The Healing Springs story is the story of the people who've lived beside South Edisto River, from the beginning of civilization to the present.

Before man set foot in this region, there was only the land, the springs, and the animals. Then the Indians migrated to the area. They drank from these springs 15,000 years before the Europeans arrived in the 1500s. From the time humans arrived there was constant change around the springs—some for the better and some for the worse.

The springs have flowed steadily, except for a brief period during the drought of 2002. Some local citizens believe the increased use of farm irrigation wells in the area has reduced the Healing Springs water flow. Throughout thousands of years animals and humans of all sizes and distinctions have drunk from the springs. This book tells the story of the springs and its inhabitants.

Raymond P. Boylston

FOREWORD

Healing Springs existed long before the first humans arrived in North America. When the springs began to flow, the land along present-day South Edisto River was quite different from what it is now. The ocean had receded for the last time leaving the landscape high and dry. Tall grass covered rolling hills and waved in the gentle breezes. Animals of all types and description, many extinct today, wandered the countryside. The skies were filled with birds of every kind flying in large flocks in all directions.

The spring water first began to flow more than a million years ago, after the Appalachian Mountains were thrust upward. Over time, mountain water accumulated, flowing under a solid layer of rock toward the ocean, increasing in pressure. A violent earthquake along present-day South Edisto River likely cracked the underground rock layer, releasing the pressurized water to the surface. It did not take long for birds and animals to find the new clear, cool springs. Traveling from all directions, they created paths to the springs. Centuries later, these paths would become trails followed by the Indians. These same trails led immigrating Europeans to the springs, where they began putting down roots, building trading posts, log cabins, and barns.

As more and more Europeans arrived and settled on farms, the native Americans grew concerned. Their hunting grounds were being taken away and they began dying by the thousands from white man's diseases. Finally they began to fight back, but it was too late. There were too many white people and the Indians were too weak. Over the centuries, they became involved in the white man's wars, fighting not only white men but other Indian tribes.

Eventually, the early European settlers, mostly English, became colonists and sought their freedom from Mother England. The Patriots and the Tories fought near the springs, where wounded redcoats were healed by drinking and bathing in the spring water. There were many skirmishes between local citizens around the time of the Revolution, especially in the South Carolina Backcountry, resulting in the first civil war in America. Once the Patriots won their freedom, they began to build their country.

South Carolina was a land of farmers, and farms surrounded the healing springs. As the population increased, there was more social contact and a need for churches. One of the first churches along the South Edisto River was Edisto Church, which later became Healing Springs Baptist Church. From that point forward, the church would be the focal point of community life. These were the years between the Revolutionary War and the Civil War. Farms had developed from a mere means of survival to a way of making profit. About the time life along the South Edisto began to improve, all hell broke loose. South Carolina seceded from the Union and the Civil War began. Many local citizens fought for the Confederacy, some losing their lives. Near the end of the conflict, the war arrived at Healing Springs. Sherman's bummers, marching from Blackville toward Columbia, marched by Healing Springs and filled their canteens with the cool water. Maybe because of the soothing effect of the water, the Federals were not so destructive around the springs as in neighboring Blackville and Barnwell. Although they took all the animals and food for miles around, they did not burn the farmhouses and barns. Once the Yankees left, everyone began rebuilding their lives. However, it would be another three months before the war ended and the survivors returned home. Slowly, year by year, things improved. By 1900, life was almost back to normal—although it would take another seventy years for the South to equal, then surpass, the North economically.

In 1944 the owner of Healing Springs, Lute Boylston, deeded the springs to Almighty God for the use of all people for all time—as it should be!

THE BEGINNING

The exact moment the springs began to flow is unknown. However, we do know that over many millions of years the landscape along the South Edisto River in South Carolina changed dramatically. Time and time again the ocean covered the land and great sheets of ice extended over much of North America. About 250 million years ago, the Appalachian Mountains were thrust upward, extending from present-day New England to the state of Georgia. This activity eventually resulted in the formation of artesian springs along the South Edisto River, one of which became known as Healing Springs.

Glacial ice sheets covered much of the Northern Hemisphere 1.7 million years ago. They began to retreat in cycles, called ice ages. Each time the ice melted, the ocean level increased covering the South Carolina Piedmont. After the final retreat of the ocean, about 20,000 years ago, rivers and streams in the region, like the Edisto River, carved permanent waterways across the Piedmont and Coastal Plain. As the climate warmed and the polar ice caps melted, large amounts of water were released into the oceans causing the sea level to rise about 300 feet. It was then the waves and currents of the inland sea eroded the land, forming an escarpment from Georgia across the midlands of South Carolina into North Carolina. This Orangeburg Escarpment resulted in the existing fall line. Excavations and wells in Barnwell County, as well as other parts of the Midlands, have revealed seashells, huge oyster shells, and prehistoric shark's teeth. Stream and river rapids above this fall line limited boat navigation. The lack of boat access was partially responsible for many of the early settlements along the fall line.

The climate in the Carolinas during ice age cycles seems to have provided a transition zone between the mountains and the coast. Cold-climate animals, such as mammoths, roamed the land with horses and other warm-climate animals. South of the glaciers, in the mid-Atlantic region, the landscape was a vast tundra. Herds of reindeer and mammoths grazed on lush vegetation in summer. During winter, these animals migrated farther south into the Carolinas. Blackville and Healing Springs are located not far from the fall line where cold-climate animals migrated.

The *Barnwell County Heritage* book, published in 1994, describes the Carolina Bays. Aerial photographs taken in the 1930s revealed a number of huge oval depressions in the earth, in North and South Carolina—some in Barnwell County, not far from Healing Springs. These depressions typically run southeast to northwest. To the south, the depressions are lined with sand; to the north, clay. One of the larger Carolina Bays, in Blackville, covers about 831 acres. With 195 sites, Barnwell County is home to one of the largest numbers of bays—one is under Heritage Trust protection. The origin of the bays is unknown, but some believe they were formed by a meteor shower millions of years ago.

The Appalachian Mountains, which formed from

wavelike folds in the earth's crust, are among the oldest mountains in the world. The range stretches about 1,500 miles. Current studies describe how these mountains, formed about 250 million years ago, were washed away and formed again about 140 million years ago. It appears, westward movement of the North American plate is still lifting the mountains. Rivers, such as the North and South forks of the Edisto, forming on the eastern side of the mountains flow into the Atlantic Ocean, while those forming on the western slopes flow into the Gulf of Mexico.

The Appalachian Mountains developed during the end of the Paleozoic Era (approximately 600 million years ago to 225 million years ago). Many times during this era, the seas flooded the Appalachian plain, including the area around Healing Springs. It was at the end of the Paleozoic, during the Permian Period, that the first seed plants, cone-bearing trees, appeared. Algae, fish, amphibians, and reptiles were plentiful. Over the next 160 million years, during the Mesozoic Era, dinosaurs, the most spectacular land animals that ever lived, ruled the earth. Approximately 65 million years ago, during the Cenozoic Era, mammals began to advance. The shallow seas drained away and the great swamplands dried up, creating better living conditions for mammals. By the middle of this era, saber-toothed cats roamed the land. Giant pigs and small horses appeared. Mammoths, mastodons, and the giant ground sloth began to arrive.

Rainwater penetrated the soil between the exposed rock layers of the Appalachian Mountains. Over millions of years, the water accumulated and ran, by force of gravity, toward the ocean. Some of the water became trapped under layers of rock, increasing in pressure as it moved seaward. One pressure point ran along South Edisto River. About 50 thousand years ago an earthquake likely cracked the underground rock layer, releasing the pressurized water. Seeking the path of least resistance to the surface, the water emerged a few miles south of South Edisto River.

The landscape where the springs emerged was similar in that time to what it is today. There were many varieties of trees and plants and numerous animals and birds. Most of the land was covered with forests of pine, oak, and cypress trees, and thick underbrush, in places, made it difficult for the animals to move. The few open spaces were caused by lightning fires. Herds of bison and mammoth grazed in the open fields. Large bears, ground sloths, saber-tooth cats, wolves, and beavers, some now extinct, also lived here.

The animals and birds quickly found the new springs and it became a favorite watering ground. As more and more animals arrived, paths were formed, leading in all directions. Each morning and afternoon a steady stream of animals used the paths to and from the springs. The first to come, just before sunrise, were the birds. There were large flocks of all descriptions, including the Carolina parakeet and carrier pigeons. As the sun rose in the east, the mammals began to appear—wolves, bears, giant sloths, deer, and, finally, bison. Instinctively, each arrived in turn. As one group finished drinking and left, the next group arrived from a different direction. There seemed to be something special about the springs.

Animals were the first to take advantage of the healing powers of the spring water. They seemed to know their wounds and ills improved after drinking or bathing in the springs. One can imagine lame and injured animals moving slowly up the paths toward the healing springs.

Life at the springs remained unchanged for about 30,000 years, until a new creature arrived—one who would change the area around the springs forever.

FIRST HUMANS

By 50,000 years ago Stone Age man had spread throughout the world. The exact time the first humans arrived in North America and how they got here is unknown. We do know that by the end of the last ice age, about 20,000 years ago, man was capable of traveling long distances by land and sea, usually following shore lines and great herds of animals they hunted. Likely, the search for animals led humans to this continent. Some of the early humans to arrive, about 15,000 years ago, followed animals over a land bridge that crossed the Bering Strait, between Alaska and Siberia. These people, no doubt a small number, traversed an ice-free corridor between the glaciers just east of the Canadian Rocky Mountains. Such bands of Stone Age men may have arrived at different periods over very long spans of time. Once they reached the lower and warmer plains, they spread across America with the animals they followed.

It is interesting to note that some of the most ancient campsites in the country are located on the East Coast. One such site, the Topper, is now being excavated near Allendale, South Carolina, about 25 miles from Healing Springs. Similar sites have been found in Cactus Hill, Virginia, and near Pittsburgh, Pennsylvania. The study of early eastern Indian skulls has revealed a strong resemblance to early Europeans. It is possible that some early Americans migrated from Europe about 20,000 years ago.

The Solutreans of Europe might have crossed the ice or come by boat across the North Atlantic, as the Vikings did 1,000 years ago. A March 2002 *National Geographic* Magazine article, "Solo Across the Arctic," described how an adventurer crossed the ice from Russia to North America in about three months.

Once in America, the first humans migrated to the warmer climates. As they settled in certain areas, such as along the Edisto River in South Carolina, their numbers greatly increased. There, they had all they needed: plenty of food, water, and means for building shelter. Evidence of early human habitation in America dating back 11,200 years was discovered in the 1920s at Clovis, New Mexico. Distinctive long spearheads, now called Clovis points, were found, along with shattered bones of bison and mammoths. Clovis points have grooves or flutes carved in the bases for attaching them to wooden shafts. Clovis points have since been found throughout North America. Humans indeed existed along with the great animals in the Ice Age.

For many years, the Clovis people were considered the first Americans. Subsequent evidence, such as that found near Allendale, South Carolina, by the Allendale Paleo-Indian Expedition of the University of South Carolina Institute of Archaeology and Anthropology, indicates that other humans arrived thousands of years earlier. Some believe these early people followed the North Atlantic sea route in kayaks.

Excavations at the Topper site in Allendale have revealed Clovis-era tools and spear points dating to 11,200 years ago. In 1998, deeper excavations revealed numerous micro stone blades, likely used by early Americans 18,000 years ago to shape wood and skin animals. Evidence of what appears to be postholes for supports to a structure, probably the oldest structure in North America, were uncovered. Sites in Pennsylvania and Virginia also revealed ancient stone tools.

This early human migration, over thousands of years, may help explain the many differences in features between native American tribes. Some were tall and others short. Skin color, facial features, skull shape, and shape of the eyes differed. Many southeastern tribes were more European in appearance than western Indians. For example, the Edisto and Cherokee were generally much taller and more slender and had lighter skin than other natives. Spanish explorer Giovanni da Verrazzano, sailing for France, wrote in 1524 that the Indians of the southeastern coastal region varied—some had broad faces while faces of those in other areas were more angular with smaller noses. Not only were there differences in appearance, but differences in language. By the time the first Europeans arrived in America, there were about 1,200 different native languages. It is believed that at least some of the variation resulted from differences in origin.

Today we know that the Healing Springs area is among the oldest inhabited areas in the Americas. Humans have been drinking the cool springs water for about 20,000 years.

NATIVE AMERICANS

The southeastern Indians enjoyed a great life prior to the arrival of the Europeans. They usually lived in small villages near sources of fresh water. Over the thousands of years of habitation, some villages located at great trading centers grew into towns with hundreds of people. One such village, called Cofitachequi, was located about thirty miles west of Healing Springs on the Savannah River at Silver Bluff. It was visited by DeSoto in 1540.

Living conditions in South Carolina were excellent—mild temperatures, sufficient rain, many animals, and numerous rivers and streams. The rivers and streams not only provided fresh water for drinking and cooking, but means of transportation in dugout canoes. As the hunters and gatherers learned to plant their own crops, the rich soil of the South Edisto River lowlands became more important.

The early Paleo-Indians, about 12,000 years ago, hunted the many animals and birds in the Southeast: mammoth, bison, deer, bears, raccoons, rabbits, beavers, opossums, squirrels, turkeys, geese, ducks, and pigeons. The numerous streams held an abundance of fish: perch, trout, catfish, and shad. The Indians fished with nets and traps. Some used spears or arrows. Fish were also caught by hand after crushed walnut husks were placed in the water to poison the fish. In some streams the water would be purposely clouded with mud, stirred up from the bottom, causing the fish to come to the surface where they were caught by hand. There was no limit to the food supply.

The many animals hunted by the Edisto not only provided food but skins for clothing, blankets, and rugs. Hides of deer, bear, beaver, and bison were used.

The southeastern Indians were among the first to begin growing their own food. Crops included maize (corn), beans, squash, melons, and pumpkins. Cultivation of food was not surprising since they and their ancestors had gathered berries, wild grapes, nuts, and various fruits for thousands of years. As the Indians observed new plants growing from seed, they began planting seed close to the villages so they would not have to travel so far to gather food. As the cultivation of food expanded, the Indians learned that the plants grew best in full sun. For the first time they had a need to clear forestland. As close observers of nature, they had seen what happened when fire burned the forest. They realized how rapidly lush new plants grew in the open ground. The Indians began to slash (cut the bark around tree trunks) and burn forests near their villages. After the trees were slashed, they died and all the foliage dropped off letting the sunshine through to the forest floor. The Indians taught the early South Carolina settlers how to slash and burn to clear land for farming. Slashed trees were often cut down, or burned down, and used to make dugout canoes.

Corn was used many ways. It was roasted in the shuck over open fires, boiled in clay pots by placing hot stones into water, ground by pounding with a wooden

15

pole on a flat rock or a burned out tree trunk, and cooked as a mush or as hominy. The dried cornhusks were used to make various things including dolls. Corn-cobs were used for fires since they release little smoke— ideal for fires inside huts.

Another source of food at various times during each year was freshwater clams. Most of the rivers and streams in the Healing Springs area were full of clams. The Indi-ans only had to wade into the water and wriggle their toes in the sandy bottom until they felt a clam. There were so many it did not take long to obtain a large quantity. A popular clamming area was the nearby Savannah River at Silver Bluff. Silver Bluff got its name because of the large number of discarded clamshells on the sides of the bluff. One of the largest shell mounds discovered is on Stallings Island in the Savannah River, near North Augusta. The mound is about 300 feet long and 300 feet wide and con-tains mussel and clam shells. Obviously, Indians gathered there to eat clams for thousands of years. Some of the old-est pottery found in North America was uncovered on Stallings Island.

The Indians learned how to treat themselves for vari-ous illnesses with plants, roots, and herbs. The medicine men knew treatments for various illnesses and they could set fractures, lance abscesses, use tourniquets, and suture wounds. They used nicotine as an antiseptic.

The results of archaeological digs at the Savannah River Site in Aiken and Barnwell Counties published in 1990 revealed numerous Indian sites along the streams there. There is no reason to believe similar Indian sites would not exist throughout the entire region, including along the South Edisto. One known site is a large Indian village located on a high bluff on the southwest bank of the South Edisto River where the Springfield-to-Williston road exits the swamp. There, in the 1930s, hundreds of arrowheads, spearheads, broken pottery, and axe heads were found by the author's brother, Sam Boylston, and his friends. On one visit to the site, Sam saw an object protruding from the ground under the porch of a farmhouse. It appeared to be the point of an arrowhead. On closer examination he found it was one of the most beautiful stone axe heads he had ever seen. There must be hundreds of similar sites all along the south (higher) bank of the South Edisto River that have never been uncovered because of underbrush and heavy tree growth. Those sites located in fields used today for farming have long been destroyed.

Many groups of Indians lived in South Carolina throughout thousands of years prior to the arrival of the Europeans. The Iroquoian Cherokee lived in the upper part of the state. They, like other Indians, traveled many miles to hunt and trade. Surely they traveled to and through Barnwell County and had contact with the Cusabo Edisto. The Siouxan Indians had tribes spread over South Carolina, including the Catawba, Waxhaw, Cheraw, Chicora, Wateree, Sampit, Sutaree, Hook, Congaree, Keyauwee, Santee, Pee Dee, Seewee, Enos, Waccamaw, and Winyaw. Many of these also had contact with the Edisto living along the South Edisto River.

Other Indians living nearby, and likely in contact with the Edisto, were the Muskogian Apalachee around the Savannah River and the Yemassee. The contact between the Edisto and the Creek living along the upper Savannah River was not so friendly. Originally the Creeks were known as the Apalachee for whom the Appalachian Mountains were named. The Chickasaw lived for a period of time near North Augusta, South Carolina. Some Notchee, expelled from Mississippi, lived in the lower part of South Carolina. Another large group of Indians was the Cusabo, with many tribes in the state, generally along the rivers. This group was important because it included the Edisto living near Healing Springs along the South Edisto River, called the Pon Pon by the Edisto Indians. The Europeans later renamed the rivers for the Indian tribes living near them. Many carry the names of the Cusabo tribes: Ashepoo, Bohickott, Coosaw, Cotachicach, Combahee, Edisto, Escamacus, Etiwan, Isaw, Kiawah, Salchichee, Stono, Wando, Wappoo, Witcheau, and Wimbee.

The Edisto and other Indians living along the South Edisto and Savannah Rivers in South Carolina during the thousands of years before the Europeans arrived were highly civilized and were exceeded in skill and knowledge only by Indians in Mexico. Due to the great number and proximity of southeastern tribes, Indians in this area tended to integrate more than elsewhere in America. In many instances one tribe would move into an area and completely replace another tribe. They knew no boundaries and freely moved where they wanted. In some cases this movement resulted in wars between tribes.

Of most importance to Indians, such as the Edisto,

living near Healing Springs, was family—following this, their tribe and then their spiritual belief. Unlike Europeans, the Edisto traced their lineage through the female side of the family. Usually, the man, once married, went to live with the wife's family. The wife's brothers and father generally trained the children. Also, the wife owned the shelter and all the furnishings. Women held an important place in the tribe and made most of the major decisions concerning the family. Some women, because of heroic acts or great accomplishments, were known as "Beloved Women"—Nancy Ward of the Cherokee is one of the better known. Children enjoyed much freedom and spent their time playing and learning to hunt and fish, plant crops, and cook. Children were often given names of animals, such as Little Fox.

Indians were very spiritual, believing in a supreme being in the sky, the source of warmth, light, and life. The sun was the symbol of the Supreme Being. They believed good and evil spirits inhabited the world. Each time an Indian killed an animal, he asked for its pardon. Each village had a medicine man or shaman who had direct contact with the spirits and engaged in elaborate ceremonies. One ceremony to purify their bodies involved brewing black drink, made like tea, from holly leaves. The drink contained caffeine and caused vomiting. Tobacco, considered a sacred plant by the Edisto and other Indians, was smoked in pipes to ward off evil, summon friendly spirits, and cure infection. It was smoked with visitors as a sign of friendliness. It was also smoked before going to war. The beautifully designed ceremonial pipes smoked by the Edisto were among their most sacred possessions. Some had carved bowls with Indian faces and animals. The French later called the peace pipe "calumet", French for flute or reed. The author found a beautiful Indian pipe bowl on the banks of the Savannah River at North Augusta, along with pieces of broken pottery. Similar finds were made at Silver Bluff, on the Savannah River, a few miles south of North Augusta.

The land, considered a sacred trust by the Indians, was the center of the universe. It was not bought or sold. Indians believed you could no more sell the land than air or the sea.

Edisto villages near Healing Springs had many lodges. The lodges were constructed of pine poles tied together with vines and leather strips. Roofs were covered with brush and straw to provide shade and protection from rain. There were both summer and winter lodges. Summer lodges had raised platforms made from logs. Straw and mats were placed on the log floors for sleeping. In winter, lodges enclosed with poles and skins were used. In the center of the lodge was a fire pit for heating and cooking. A hole in the roof above the fire pit let the smoke escape. Usually, raised platforms lining the sides of the lodges were used for sleeping and sitting. Each section of the lodge, assigned to individuals in the family, was decorated with that individual's personal items. Villages usually had a hot house where water was poured over hot rocks to create a sauna effect for cleansing and treating illnesses.

Most large villages had a public square in the center. Lodges and storage sheds for grain were situated around it. The chief's lodge was positioned in the best location, close to, but apart from, the others. Near the chief's lodge was a council house where tribal meetings were held. As villages grew, temple mounds were built. Some large villages had celebration and ball fields.

Most Indian celebrations and ceremonies were associated with the seasons of the year. The Green Corn Ceremony, for example, a thanksgiving celebration, occurred in July or August, depending on the harvest for that year. When the corn ripened and was ready for harvest, the large villages sent runners to other villages announcing the Green Corn Ceremony was to take place. To ensure all villages knew the exact day of the ceremony, the runners gave a bundle of short sticks to each village chief. A stick was to be removed and broken each day until the last stick was broken, indicating it was time to travel to the ceremony. Each group of Indians took gifts and food with them, since the ceremony lasted about eight days.

During the first three days the men drank the black drink to cleanse themselves of evil spirits. Then all fires were extinguished except the one sacred fire. A new fire was prepared. Small sticks were placed in the center of four logs, which formed a cross. The medicine man started the new fire by twirling a fire drill and praying. As the fire caught and burned, the logs were pushed inward with an ear of corn on each log. The medicine man, usually dressed in white buckskin with white buckskin moccasins, removed the ears of corn from the logs and placed them in the fire as an offering of thanksgiving for the harvest. When all the corn was burned, each family lit a fire from the new sacred fire. After lighting their fires, the families danced and played games for five days. At the conclusion of the games, an orator, usually one of the tribal leaders, would speak to the people urging them to remain true to their ancient customs.

It is interesting to note that the idea of a perpetual fire and an annual festival to extinguish the old fire and ignite a new one was practiced by ancient Europeans. The first humans from ancient Europe likely brought this custom with them to America.

There were a number of games played by the Indians. One such game, described by Virginia Pounds Brown and Laurella Owens in their book *The World of Southern Indians*, was "chunkey" involving two players. One player started the game by rolling a smooth stone disk, about five inches in diameter and one-half inch thick, down a flat, rectangular playing field. Both players then raced after the Chunkey stone with eight-foot poles sharpened at the ends. The object of the game was to throw the javelin-like poles as close to the spot where the stone disk would stop rolling. The player throwing his pole nearest to the stone disk made one point—two points if he struck the disc. There was much betting among the onlookers.

The Indians played a ball game similar to lacrosse, with as many as 100 players on each side. Often these games were played against distant tribes and are believed to have substituted for war. There were only a few rules, like remaining inside a specific boundary. Some fields had very large boundaries, extending over a mile. It was a rough and tumble game resulting in many serious injuries and some deaths. Like a battle, those injured or killed were honored.

An Indian family usually arranged a marriage once a young man became attracted to a young woman and the woman agreed to the union. Marriages were not approved between individuals within the same family. A husband or wife could end a marriage by simply moving out. Premarital sex was not condoned and individuals caught in the practice were usually punished. While most marriages were monogamous, some wealthy men had several concubines.

Indians tended to have happy childhoods as their parents and relatives were indulgent. Physical punishment was rare and considered unnecessary to correct any problem. Young boys spent most of their time learning necessary skills for adulthood such as trailing, tracking, stalking, shooting, hunting, fishing, and swimming. Young girls stayed close to home with their mother, grandmother, and aunts, learning to plant, cultivate, harvest, tend fires, make clothing, and cook.

Indians liked to dance and usually did so at every opportunity—festivals, weddings, rites, and preparation for war.

As a general rule, Indian tribes, like the Edisto, practiced democracy. Most major tribal decisions were made by the council, composed of elders with representatives from each village clan. Both men and women served as council members and enjoyed the right to speak, which they did with eloquence. Each item brought before the council was discussed before a vote was taken. The ceremonial pipe passed from member to member clockwise around the council. Blowing a puff of smoke upward along the pipe stem indicated an affirmative vote. Not smoking the pipe indicated a negative vote.

The council always voted on whether to go to war against another tribe. In most cases, warfare was more of a show than actual strife. It was conducted with ceremony and there were few deaths. The swift raids were made by small war parties usually in retaliation to a previous attack. Such raids gave young men a chance to prove their bravery and older warriors a chance to show their leadership skills. Success in battle depended on how well they conducted their prewar ceremonies, which lasted about three days. During this ceremony they drank the black drink and painted their bodies. They danced and sang chants.

Preparing to leave, each strapped on his back a deerskin pack containing a blanket, a leather pouch of parched corn, cornmeal, and a wooden cup or small gourd. Each carried a bow and arrows, a stone-bladed knife, and a club in his belt. The clubs were often spiked with imbedded teeth and used in hand-to-hand fighting. Some warriors also carried a cane shield. Villagers stood along the trail encouraging the warriors along as they left on their mission.

Once the raiding party entered enemy territory, they moved quietly on moccasined feet. Surprise was crucial to the success of the raid. They had to be as close as possible to the enemy village before launching their attack. To confuse the enemy and avoid detection, they often divided their small band into two groups, each group approaching in single file from different directions. Communication between each group, when necessary, was by predesignated animal calls. If they succeeded in their surprise, the raid ended quickly. The attackers often simply touched an enemy with special sticks. Such acts were considered as brave as killing an enemy. Objects would be taken from the enemy village and carried home as trophies. In some cases, women, young girls, and children were kidnapped.

After returning home following a successful raid, villagers celebrated for about three days, singing, dancing, and feasting. Young men participating in their first raid were given special names and the right to wear certain feathers.

Indians were keen observers of nature and animals. Soon after the first humans arrived near Healing Springs, they would certainly have observed the numerous animal trails leading to and from the artesian springs. As it was a good area to hunt, the Indians frequented the springs. Surely, they saw that many of the animals drinking from the springs were injured, lame, or ill. Returning to their village, the hunters would have told the medicine man about what they saw. In turn, the medicine man would have had the hunters lead him to the springs where he too saw ill and lame animals. Tasting the clear, cool water flowing like a fountain from the ground, the medicine man, legend tells us, began to sing, chant, and dance around. He then declared the springs a sacred gift of the Great Spirit to heal the sick and lame. He warned that from that time forward there must be no killing of animals at the healing springs and the spring water be consumed only by the sick and injured.

Despite the European image of the Indians as savage and warlike, most were peaceful and, in some respects, more civilized than the Europeans.

Over the thousands of years prior to the arrival of Europeans in South Carolina, Indian tribes moved into and out of the Healing Springs area. One group during the Mississippian Period built large earthen mounds, usually along rivers. Many of these mounds still exist today—some stand eighty feet tall. The mound builders surrounded their villages with wooden palisades and often set up maze-like entrances. Wide ditches were dug around the palisades. Tribesmen's farms were located outside the village, but nearby. Flint tied to oak handles were hoes used for chopping weeds and planting. Shells and flattened wood were also used as hoes. During this period Indian agriculture improved and they were able to accumulate food surpluses. These surpluses were stored inside raised sheds in pottery, which had improved in quality and quantity. The mound builders disappeared about the time the first Europeans arrived in America.

Rumors spread throughout the southeastern Indian tribes about white people sailing and landing on the coast of Florida. They arrived, it was said, in big dugouts from across the ocean. Some Indians reported fights with the white men who used fire sticks to kill attacking Indians. Most Indians living in South Carolina expected that someday they would see these new strangers.

In the early 1500s Spanish explorers visited Mexico and then Florida. The Calusa Indians of Florida were the first southeastern native Americans to meet the Spanish Europeans. These first encounters were not all friendly. Ponce de Leon returned to Florida in 1513. Then in 1539, Hernando De Soto began exploring the Southeast with 600 well-armed soldiers, slaves, and servants; 24 Catholic priests; and 220 horses, pigs, mules, and bloodhounds. Indians in Georgia told De Soto about the great, wealthy Indian city of Cofitachequi located on the Savannah River.

EUROPEANS

The first Europeans to set foot on South Carolina soil were Spanish explorers sent out by Lucas Vasquez de Ayllon in 1514 and again in 1521. They landed on present-day Pawley's Island in 1521. The Chicora, who at first were afraid of the bearded white men, greeted them. The Spanish gained the trust of the natives by offering them gifts. In turn, the Indians helped the Spanish explore the countryside. After the Spanish got what they wanted, they turned on the Indians.

In 1521, the Spanish invited 140 Chicora aboard their ship. Once on board, the Indians were detained and taken to Hispaniola where they were sold as slaves. Thus began the slave trade in America.

The Spanish established the first European settlement in South Carolina in 1526. As more and more Europeans arrived, the Indians' suffering increased. Their hunting grounds were taken and they began to contract the white man's diseases.

As De Soto's expedition moved northward from Florida in 1539, the Spaniards spread terror among the Indians in their path. De Soto's men used crossbows and guns to kill many natives. Large dogs attacked and frightened them. Indians soon began to send runners ahead of the Spanish party to warn other tribes. The Indians at Cofitachequi and the Edisto knew of the white man's coming long before their arrival. They held a council meet-

ing and discussed their options. The decision was made
not to attack the strangers but offer friendship and food.
Many Indian tribes, for miles around Silver Bluff, sent representatives to meet and learn about the strangers.

Cofitachequi had once been one of the largest and
wealthiest Indian cities north of Mexico. Over the centuries prior to the European migration, Cofitachequi had
begun to decline, for reasons unknown. Despite this
trend, the great city still enjoyed a large population and
and much wealth. The Indians in Georgia knew this and
sent De Soto to the city in search of wealth.

At the time of De Soto's arrival in present-day Aiken
County, about 30 miles miles from Healing Springs,
Cofitachequi was ruled by an elderly woman. Upon learning of De Soto's approach, villagers moved their ruler to
safety. The old woman's niece, Cacica Perico, was designated to represent the city. Over half the people living in
the city went away with the old woman. Those who remained were delegated to watch the Spanish and be prepared to fight if necessary, but to avoid battle if at all possible.

Cacica and her entourage waited for De Soto on the
high bluff on the South Carolina side of the Savannah
River. At the foot of the bluff a number of canoes waited,
ready for launch. When De Soto arrived on the Georgia
side of the Savannah River, Cacica climbed into a large
canoe shaded by canopy while her men boarded the other
canoes. Braves paddled across the wide river. The young
woman's stately demeanor impressed the Spanish, who
called her La Senora de (the lady of) Cofitachequi. Upon

reaching the Georgia shore, Cacica was assisted from her canoe by her attendants.

Cacica stood straight and confident. Her beautiful clothes were adorned with colorful beads. A string of freshwater pearls, the size of hazelnuts, circled her neck three times and hung down to her thighs. As she approached De Soto, Cacica removed the pearls and placed the string around the Spaniard's neck. In response, De Soto presented her with a ruby ring from his finger.

After the greeting, De Soto's men and belongings were transported across the Savannah River in the Indian canoes. Once they arrived at Cofitachequi, the Spanish were provided lodges and food. That evening the visitors were invited to a feast in the city square. During the feast, the Indians presented the Spanish with deerskins. The Spaniards let the Indians know what they really wanted was gold and silver. The Indians then brought out copper and iron pyrite, which did not impress the Spanish.

Realizing what the Spanish sought, the young woman led De Soto to a sacred lodge where the bones of her ancestors lay. There, large baskets overflowed with hundreds of pounds of large freshwater pearls. Surely, De Soto's eyes must have popped at the sight. Records indicate the explorers carried away over 350 pounds of pearls.

The Cofitachequi Indians are said to have been clothed in tanned deer hides of superior quality. They wore pants, buckskins, and black garters laced with white hide, all fringed in colored hide. Warriors wore breastplates and leather helmets and used hide shields. The villagers were elegant, civilized, and well-mannered. The

Spaniards questioned the Indians about the buffalo hides. The buffalo, which roamed the North American plains, were unknown to the Europeans.

The temple lodge at Cofitachequi stood on a high mound. The large structure was decorated with beautiful mats. Situated around the temple lodge were about 500 smaller lodges for housing and storage. The roofs of the lodges and temple were covered with layers of split cane, tightly woven. The large temple doors were flanked on each side by twelve carved wooden figures. Inside the temple, rows of benches near the floor held painted wooden chests with the bones of the city's royalty. Other containers held pearls, skins, and cloth. Eight large rooms surrounding the inner temple contained weapons and tools such as clubs, axes, and picks, as well as shields of buffalo hide.

De Soto's men described open forests of walnut and mulberry trees and fertile fields surrounding the great Indian city. They unearthed a metal dagger and false pearls belonging to Vasquez de Ayllon's expedition, evidence of earlier contact between Indians and Europeans.

During their stay, De Soto and his men were well treated. The Spaniards returned the natives' friendship and good will by stealing, torturing, and raping. Preparing to leave, De Soto, as he had done in other villages on his route, captured the ruler's young niece who was allowed to take some of her servants. The Indians were forced to show the Spaniards the trails northward toward the mountains. After about three weeks, the young woman and her attendants escaped and returned to Cofitachequi. De Soto continued his trip to the west where he died at the Mississippi River in Louisiana in 1542. About 300 of De Soto's men survived the expedition.

The Healing Springs Indians returned home after De Soto left Cofitachequi. They told of the evil Spaniards and how they had kidnapped the young woman despite her friendship. Little did they know this was just the beginning of cruelty by white men against all native Americans. Juan Pardo, a member of De Soto's party, returned to the city about twenty-six years later and reported it was then only a small village.

In 1560, Tristan de Luna led another Spanish expedition, tracing De Soto's route through the Southeast. The explorers learned that a sick Spanish slave left behind by De Soto had started an epidemic that spread through the Coosa Indians, decimating the population. A similar series of epidemics virtually wiped out all southeastern Indian tribes.

French Huguenots established a settlement on the South Carolina coast in 1562. The next year, French artist Jacques Le Moyne began drawing some of the first pictures of South Carolina Indians. In 1566, the Spanish attacked and destroyed the settlement.

As the 1600s began, Europeans invaded America from all directions, driving the Indians from their hunting grounds. The Spanish attacked from the south and southwest, the French from the north down the St. Lawrence and Mississippi Rivers, the English and Dutch from the east, and the Russians down the west coast. In general, the Indians encountered by the Europeans were humane. Despite this, the natives were viewed as savages, an uncivilized wilderness people, prime candidates for subjection.

TRADERS AND SETTLERS

During the period 1630–1642 there was a great migration of settlers from England to Massachusetts. Over 16,000 Englishmen, discontented with the Anglican Church and the government under King Charles I, decided to come to America and start new lives. Many of the parents of original settlers around Healing Springs, South Carolina, were among these New England colonists, including the author's Boylston ancestors.

One of the first Englishmen to live among the South Carolina Indians and learn their ways was Dr. Henry Woodward in 1666. He likely had contact with the Indians living near Healing Springs. While Woodward was living with the Indians, the English settled Charles Town. Settler Maurice Matthews wrote Lord Ashley Cooper, "The Indians all about us are friends." He described his trip to the upper reaches of the Ashley River in May of 1671: "About thirty miles or more upward, we came among the Cusso Indians, our friends. . . ." About a month later, the Grand Council of the Colony of Carolina declared war on the Cusso (Edisto), alleging they stole grain and livestock from the settlers. The revenge of the English settlers must have been sure and swift, as the Council recorded on October 2, 1671, ". . . said Indians had been disposed of and the captured Indians would be transported to the West Indies as slaves." However, the Council did allow the remaining Cusso to give themselves up, make peace, and purchase the captured Indians back with deerskin. This likely initiated one of the largest deerskin trading businesses in America.

While the early missionaries in South Carolina, including Dr. Woodward, and the fur traders were friendly to the Indians for obvious reasons, the Indians considered most settlers their enemies. The settlers moved in and began clearing the land, and the Indians felt challenged. Many Europeans regarded the Indians as "vermin" to be exterminated along with other wild animals in the forest, as evidenced by colonial legislatures authorizing rewards for Indian scalps and selling Indians as slaves.

According to historians, in the late 1600s the second English settlement was established at a bend in the Edisto River near the South Carolina coast. This frontier town, called New London, was settled by religious dissenters. All evidence of New London has vanished, but a plat from about 1700 reveals a village of approximately 500 acres and 250 lots—80 homes, multiple stores, a school, a church, a blacksmith's shop, and a barber shop.

Ownership of land was the main source of conflict between Indians and settlers. The Indians did not recognize private ownership of land. The easiest course of action for the Europeans to take in dealing with this problem was to eliminate the contenders. And that's what they did. The white man's diseases, however, did more to eradicate the Indians than conflict over land. Smallpox epidemics almost wiped out some tribes. In 1705, to avoid the further spread of disease, Pennsylvania's legislature passed a law against "the further importation of Indian slaves from Carolina."

It is important to understand that the Indians had lived in America almost as long as the Europeans had lived in Europe. America was their home. Indians attacked settlers because the settlers took their hunting grounds. They were defending their home against invaders, as the people of any country defend against invaders. Mistreatment on both sides continued for more than one hundred years—until the native Americans were finally overcome by the much larger immigrating force.

During the late 1600s and early 1700s, many Indians displaced by the European settlers joined with their neighboring tribes. This blending of tribes has made it very difficult to trace individual tribes, such as the Edisto. This blending also resulted in a mix of languages. Of all the Indian tribes living in the southeastern woodlands, only the languages of the five so-called "civilized tribes"—Cherokee, Creek, Choctaw, Chickasaw, and Seminole—remain today.

Dr. Woodward, who lived among the Indians, left the Robert Sanford expedition in 1666 to join the Edistos, trading places with a brave called "Shadoo" as a sort of cultural exchange program. Robert Sanford, leader of the expedition through South Carolina stated, "I put into the river [Edisto] again and being anchored went ashore on the East point of the entrance, where I found Shadoo [Chief of the Edisto, who had been with Hilton at Barbados]. He and several other Indians came from the town by land to see our coming. I asked whether this was the river, which Hilton was in. They told me no, that it was

36

the next river. I demanded the name of the river. They told me 'Edistowe.'"

It became obvious to the English settlers at Charles Town in the late 1600s that much money could be made by trading with the Indians for deerskins. There were hundreds of thousands of deer throughout the colony and the Indians had been killing them for thousands of years. The settlers proposed a trade. Rather than merely hunting deer for food and clothing for their families, the Indians would hunt in exchange for white man's items. With this deal, the entire culture and future of the Indians would change for the worse, as the traders gave the Indians little of value, such as beads, in return.

Deerskins formed the core of the fur trade in South Carolina. By 1700, many traders were pushing far into the Backcountry. It has been estimated that, at the turn of the century, about 70,000 skins were shipped from Charleston annually. By 1731, the number was up to 225,000 each year. This tremendous business opportunity was the initial incentive for Backcountry, or westward, expansion and settlement. Eventually, this expansion resulted in conflicts between the Indians and English settlers, between the English and French, as well as the Spanish. In the conflicts Indians took sides among settlers and fought each other.

Exploration of the South Carolina Backcountry was relatively easy for the initial traders as there were numerous Indian trails, which had existed for thousands of years. A trader would load his merchandise and supplies in packs and place them on one or two mules. Carrying his musket on his shoulder and leading his mules, he began his long walk into the wilderness. Hardly a day passed that he did not meet with Indians. At night he camped on high ground near a stream and cooked his meal. After eating, he rolled out his blanket and slept on the ground, usually with the reins of his mules tied to his arm. The next morning he continued his trip until finding an Indian village where he would begin negotiating for deerskin. Often he remained in the village for some time, as long as the Indians continued to bring in deerskins. Trading posts were eventually established at locations where deerskins were plentiful.

One of the first traders to the Healing Springs area of the Backcountry was Nathaniel Walker, reputedly born May 12, 1724, in England, likely of Irish descent. He was in the Waxhaws in the mid 1700s, south of present-day Charlotte, North Carolina, in Craven County on land granted by the Royal Order of King George III. He married a cousin from Virginia. The couple's oldest son was also called Nathaniel.

Like most early colonists, the Walkers moved often, looking for better opportunities. After leaving the Waxhaws, he and his family lived at Cane Creek, near Lynches Creek. On occasion, he filled in as preacher for wilderness churches. In 1755, while in the Lynches Creek area, he met Reverend James Smart. Smart later moved with some of his followers to the Coosawhatchie area. It is believed that Walker visited Smart and was captivated by the beautiful, fertile region along the South Edisto River and decided to relocate his family about 40 miles up the South Edisto, near Healing Springs. There, about

1757, he established his home and a trading post near the friendly Edisto Indians. The plat for Nathaniel Walker's land places the property south of the South Edisto River on Windy Hill Creek in Orangeburg District.

Not long after Nathaniel Walker moved to the Healing Springs area he made contact with Indians living a few miles from his trading post on the river and began trading with them. It is likely that one day, while hunting, he headed down a well-used trail, rife with animal and Indian tracks. As he moved toward the southeast, the trail led into a clump of trees. He approached the trees quietly and cautiously. Upon entering the shadow of the trees he paused to let his eyes adjust. Then he slowly moved forward. After walking a few yards, he saw some movement. He cocked his flintlock so he would be ready to fire his musket quickly, if necessary. Just then he saw an old Indian drinking from a pool of water. The elder was on his knees dipping water with his hands. Hearing someone behind him, the Indian rose suddenly and moved away from the water. Approaching, Walker recognized the local Edisto Indian chief. After they greeted, the chief led Walker to the artesian springs, explaining that they were considered sacred by his people, as the water had healing power and only the sick and injured were allowed to drink from the springs. Walker was intrigued and wondered how he might acquire the property. The old Indian chief went on to say that the springs were owned by the Great Spirit and could not be bought or sold. The chief told Walker, however, that he could use the springs in exchange for trade goods. Of course, Walker concluded he was purchasing the springs. Such was the case for many so called "purchases" from Indians.

News of the healing springs spread through the community. Soon settlers were trekking to the springs to drink the water. They were not sure if it healed but they all concluded the water was some of the best tasting they had ever drunk. Their trips to the springs would become routine.

As more and more settlers moved into the Backcountry, Walker's trading post became a traveler's rest and stagecoach stop along the old Charles Town-to-Augusta road. Walker began to serve as a surveyor for the Commissioner of Locations. As such, he knew everyone moving into the area.

Most of the early Backcountry houses were crude, temporary shelters made from pine logs with split shingle roofs. The floors were dirt and chimneys built of local stone and dried clay mud. Clay mud was also used to chink between the logs in the walls. The early cabins were soon replaced with more permanent board frame and clapboard side houses raised off the ground with wooden floors. Most homes had a central hall running from front to back, flanked by two rooms on each side. The kitchen was detached, with a connecting covered porch, for fire safety and to reduce the heat in summer.

Each family had at least one member who could build simple wooden furniture of poplar, cypress, walnut, oak, and pine. Due to a lack of room, dining tables were not left standing, but were leaned against the wall when not in use. Few chairs were made and those usually for the head of the house. Most family members sat on benches or stools.

Some of the new Healing Springs settlers in the late 1750s were frontier families from Pennsylvania, Virginia, and North Carolina. Many were trying to escape the Cherokee Indian attacks during the French and Indian War, which lasted from 1754 to 1763. There were a number of Indian attacks in South Carolina during this war. In 1760, a Cherokee war party attacked a refugee wagon train mired in a swamp near Long Cane Creek. John C. Calhoun's grandmother was killed in the attack.

Settlers living in remote areas that could not be defended against attacks by the Cherokee moved to safety, usually stopping at trading posts such as Walker's near Healing Springs. There they raised palisades and fortified houses. The British sent out expeditions against the Indians in 1760 and 1761. The second expedition met the Cherokee in June at the battle of Etchohik, near the town of Edistowe and routed them. The British then burned all the Cherokee villages they could find as well as the Indians' crops and orchards. About 5,000 Cherokee were driven into the mountains. In turn, the Cherokees asked for peace. A conference was held in Augusta, Georgia, in 1763 where representatives of the southeastern Indian tribes met and established a line along the frontier the colonists were not to cross. White settlers soon forgot this agreement.

During the French and Indian War, there was much unrest in the Backcountry. The local provincial militia felt they were left alone in most cases to fight for their lives, families, and homes without assistance from Charles Town. Vigilante groups formed. As refugees ran from the Indians, some moved onto property abandoned by others. After the war was over, the refugees tried to keep the lands they occupied. Squatters, poachers, and thieves were a real problem, but the greatest threat was from organized gangs of outlaws roaming the Backcountry.

By 1766, a crime wave was sweeping through the Carolina Backcountry. Settler farms experienced sudden attacks by gangs of outlaws on horseback. Farmers were sometimes captured and tortured and the outlaws held red-hot pokers against the farmers' feet in an effort to learn where valuables were hidden. Women and young girls suffered kidnap and rape.

Trading posts, such as Walker's, were especially vulnerable because of supplies stored there. Such locations were often built like small forts so they could be defended. If the outlaws managed to capture a trading post owner, they demanded a ransom, threatening to burn the post to the ground if it wasn't paid. In most cases, the local militia were too few and too widespread to provide much protection. Occasionally, an outlaw was captured and sent under armed guard to Charles Town. In one case, eleven outlaws were hauled before the court in Charles Town. Only six were convicted and the other five received pardon from the governor. This outcome did not sit well with the Backcountry's law-abiding citizens who had been terrorized for months.

In 1767, Backcountry men, including those around Healing Springs, concluded that if the government in

Charles Town wouldn't protect them, they would protect themselves. Communities began to pool their resources and turn on the outlaw gangs. These vigilantes located and attacked outlaw hideouts, capturing many of the culprits and hanging them. Learning of this action, the government in Charles Town ordered the citizens to disband.

Upon receiving the order, the vigilantes formed a unit called the Regulators. The Regulators represented all the South Carolina Backcountry and fought to insure that the Charles Town government sent law enforcement officials to serve in the Backcountry like those in the Lowcountry. The Regulators numbered about 3,000, including those from around Healing Springs and Orangeburg. Most were small farmers who owned around 100 acres of land apiece. Each region had a captain. At Healing Springs, Nathaniel Walker held that honor.

The Regulators petitioned the Charles Town government for courts, courthouses, jails, and schools. As a result, the Charles Town Assembly authorized two companies of rangers to be sent into the Backcountry to restore order. The mounted ranger companies successfully drove the outlaws away. Of those captured, sixteen were hanged in North Carolina. Others were sent to Charles Town for trial. In 1768, circuit courts were established in the interior.

Although the outlaw gangs had been dissolved, criminals still roamed the Backcountry. Because of this continual threat, the Regulators refused to disband and met in a congress near present-day Columbia where they adopted a formal plan of Regulation. The Regulators were

43

clearly in control of all South Carolina Backcountry—from fifty miles inland of the Atlantic to the mountains. For about three years the Backcountry functioned separately from the Lowcountry, achieving the law and order they sought.

Some Regulators, however, took advantage of the situation for their own gain. Prominent Backcountry men and farmers around Orangeburg organized against the Regulators and soon formed a local Moderator Militia. They assembled along the Bush and Saluda Rivers near present-day Columbia and were ready to battle the Regulators when a truce was signed. This truce ended the Regulator movement in South Carolina and allowed Backcountry settlers to begin returning their lives to normal.

EARLY HEALING SPRINGS SETTLERS

Many settlers arrived in the South Carolina Backcountry from Charles Town. Many more came down the Great Wagon Road, which ran from Harrisburg, Pennsylvania, through the Shenandoah Valley of Virginia, into the Carolinas. This road ran through Cherokee country and travel often resulted in conflicts with the Indians. Over the years the English negotiated alliances with Backcountry Indians to serve as a buffer against more hostile tribes, which included the Westo, the Creek, and the Savannah. These alliances often failed, as friendly Indians became hostile and hostile Indians became friendly.

Despite the unrest with the Indians and the unlawfulness in the Backcountry, the period from 1725 to 1775 was one of great public and private prosperity. Once the Backcountry settlers achieved a level of self-sufficiency, they began to seek ways to make a profit. Some of these early profit crops were hemp and indigo, which could result in profits of $27,000 for a good growing season. Getting their harvest to market was not easy. The South Edisto and Savannah Rivers were usually used for transport.

Besides the Indians, the greatest threat to the early South Carolina settlers was disease, which was more prevalent here than in other colonies. Between 1670 and 1775, South Carolina had fifty-nine major epidemics, including eighteen yellow fever, nine smallpox, and four influenza. Malaria was also epidemic, especially in the Lowcountry, and was fatal to young children and pregnant women. Childhood mortality rates may have reached eighty percent. Most families had their own burial grounds on their farms. Because of the wooden grave markers used, most of these early graveyards have been lost.

Settlers moving into the Healing Springs area brought their belongings on their backs, on mules, and, in some cases, in wagons. Once settled on their land, they used the trees on their property to build simple log cabins. The first homes and barns often had dirt floors. Some logs were sawed by hand into short sections and split into wooden shingles. Due to the heat in South Carolina, most cabins had covered porches. There was a shortage of skilled labor, expensive nails, and glass. Since these early log cabins were placed directly on the ground, most have been lost to decay. A few cabins placed on stone or log blocks survived for many years.

Cabin doors swung on wooden hinges and had wooden latches. A door often had a slot cut in it for observing outside and firing weapons. Kitchens, barns, and smokehouses stood detached from the main house. Near the cabins were open fields for gardens and crops. Newcomers learned from the local Indians and other settlers how to slash and burn the forest to clear the land. They also learned what and how to plant.

Mattresses were stuffed with straw, later with feathers, and placed on wooden beds. Cradles and trundle beds for children were stored under large beds. Other furnishings included trunks, chests, chests of drawers, food safes, and cupboards made of walnut, maple, oak, and pine.

The kitchen was the principal place for gathering as a family. Initially, the chimneys were made of logs and dried clay. Later, local rocks and finally bricks were used. Fireplaces were very large to accommodate the iron pots and kettles. Pots swung on iron rods over the fire for cooking. Iron tongs, shovels, pans, racks, andirons, and skillets served as cooking utensils. Families ate their meals at the kitchen table using wooden or metal plates, knives, and forks. Some pewter and earthenware plates were used.

Wild animals, birds, and fish supplied the meat they needed. Once settled and able to do so, a farmer purchased and raised pigs, cows, ducks, chickens, sheep, and goats. They planted orchards of apples, peaches, pears, pecans, walnuts, and plums. The fruit was not only used for baking and eating raw but also to make liquor. At weddings and funerals, settlers usually drank coffee, tea, sassafras tea, and apple cider.

These were hardworking people who rose early in the morning and worked until dark. Getting up about daybreak they built a fire in the fireplace and put on a pot of coffee. Grabbing a quick snack, like a biscuit with a small piece of cured ham left over from the day before, they set off outside to begin their morning chores. They drew water from the well or spring, fed the livestock, and milked the cow. If there were older children in the family, they helped with the chores.

The women got up with the men. They made the bed and began to prepare breakfast. One of the first things to go on the fire was an iron pot of water for grits. As the grits cooked, bacon was sliced from a side of salt cured pork and placed in an iron skillet with water. The skillet was placed on an iron rack over the burning coals and brought to a boil to remove most of the salt. Then the water was poured off and the bacon fried. By then the aroma filled the small kitchen. Flour was dipped from a barrel in the corner and placed in a large wooden bowl. Soda, lard, and buttermilk were added to the flour and mixed in by hand. Once the right consistency was reached, the dough was placed on a floured board and kneaded. The dough was then rolled out flat and pieces were pinched off and patted out by hand. The biscuits were placed in a Dutch oven resting on the coals in the fireplace. Using a small iron shovel with a long wooden handle, hot coals were placed on the lid of the Dutch oven. As the biscuits baked, the bacon was removed from the skillet and placed on a plate. Fresh eggs were fried in the bacon grease.

By this time, the children were up and dressed. After making their beds and washing their faces and hands in a washbasin on the back porch, they entered the kitchen like hungry bear cubs. A farm bell or an iron triangle with a metal rod, hanging on the back porch, was rung to signal the men and older children to breakfast. Usually this was between 8 and 9 A.M. Meals, such as breakfast, were the only times the entire family was together to talk and share.

Often there was no lunch, except for a cold snack and well water. Dinner, called supper, was usually during late afternoon, after the fieldwork was over. Biscuits, cornbread, or hoecakes were served, along with fried ham or chicken. Available vegetables from the garden, potatoes, and fruit were prepared. During the summer, women baked pies using wild blackberries. Sugar cane syrup was on the table at each meal and often sopped with biscuits. Once the settlers obtained a cow, buttermilk and butter were also available. Clabber was made from milk and eaten like yogurt or sour cream. On Sundays and special occasions, rice was cooked. Very little beef was eaten.

Except for the fireplace, a settler's other primary light source was a crude Betty Lamp, which was a wick in a small saucer of oil. When needed, candles were used. By the late 1700s, most settlers were using improved lamps made of pewter and glass.

Most everyday clothing worn by Healing Springs farmers was homemade. Each house had a spinning wheel and a set of hand cards for drawing out and aligning the cotton or wool fibers. Flax was also used to make Irish linen. Handlooms, similar to those of the Indians, were used to make clothes. The oldest children often did the spinning. If a girl did not marry, she became the "spinster" of the family.

There was the constant threat of sickness among the settlers. Most Europeans contracted malaria (ague) soon after arriving in South Carolina. In 1756, the Anglican congregation of St. Philips Parish in Charles Town recorded 105 deaths, 35 of whom were children under 3 years old. Only a few people lived into their eighties. There was one doctor for every 600 colonists in South

Carolina.

Springs, creeks, streams, and rivers have always been an important part of life in the Healing Springs and Blackville area. The two greatest bodies of water are the South Edisto River and the Savannah River. These rivers were some of the earliest means of transportation into and out of the South Carolina Backcountry. Of the two rivers, the South Edisto played a more direct role in the lives of the local inhabitants. The Edisto is one of the longest black water rivers in the world. The dark brown water, which appears black, derives its color from decayed leaves in the swamps along the river. Underground springs feeding the river keep the water fresh and cool. Some of the best-tasting fish in South Carolina come from the South Edisto. These include largemouth bass, red breast, and catfish. Those who eat catfish stew made with fresh South Edisto River catfish never forget the experience.

There are numerous streams around Healing Springs and Blackville: Sheepford Creek, Snake Creek, Little Salkehatchie Creek, Toby Creek, Turkey Creek, Reeves Creek, and Windy Hill Creek. These creeks supplied water for prehistoric animals, Indians, and settlers. In the 1700s some of the streams were dammed to form ponds for sawmills and gristmills. Generations of Indians and settlers and their descendants have enjoyed skinny-dipping in the cool streams.

Many of the original artesian springs throughout the area have ceased flowing. Healing Springs continued to flow until the drought of 2002, when the water slowed to a trickle and finally stopped. As soon as the rainfall increased and the underground water supply was replenished, the springs began flowing again. Once more, vehicles of all descriptions waited in a long line so the people inside could fill plastic jugs and buckets with the healing water.

Early settlers tried to purchase land on rivers and other waterways for easy personal travel and transportation of farm products to market. There were both public and private landings, like Boylston Landing on the South Edisto River near Healing Springs, belonging to the author's family. Small and large dugout canoes and larger flat-bottom boats were used. In transporting timber, logs were tied together and floated down the rivers to Charles Town and Savannah for sale.

Although there were some roads, these were rough, muddy, and dusty. Most roads followed the old Indian trails and footpaths, which were originally animal paths. Homes and farms were connected to the main roads by bridle paths. Causeways made of logs placed in the direction of road travel and then covered with mud and dirt crossed the numerous South Carolina swamps. Smaller tree limbs were then overlaid on top of the dirt to form a firm surface. These causeways led to and from ferry landings. The ferries were flat-bottom boats tied to a large rope strung across the river. Poles and paddles or pulleys were used to move the ferryboats across. Most of the ferry landings later became bridge locations.

It was not only difficult to travel through the swamps but also through the countryside. Many roads, rounded to ensure the rain run off, became slippery in clay areas. It

was not unusual for horses, mules, and wagons to slide
into ditches. Roads through deep sand made for slow
travel. The narrow roads held the additional threat of
dead trees falling across and striking wagons, horses, and
people. Many early travelers described in letters and memoirs how lonely and dull travel was through the South
Carolina Backcountry. A traveler could ride or walk an
entire day through sandy pine barrens and dismal swamps
without seeing another person or a house. Because of the
difficulties, most early settlers traveled no more than fifty
miles from their birthplaces in a lifetime. Also, the poor
transportation system meant poor communications. However, there were some newspapers and regular postal service by the late 1700s.

Healing Springs settlers in the 1700s were generally of
English and Scots-Irish descent. A few were Swiss-German.
Some Scots had fled Scotland after the English defeat of
the Highlanders at the Battle of Cullodin in April 1746.
Others were Scots-Irish sent to Northern Ireland by James
I in an effort to replace the hostile Catholic Irish. Due to
overpopulation in Northern Ireland, many Scots-Irish,
such as the Reeds, were encouraged to settle in America.
This was an independent, self-reliant religious group, with
strong love of home and family. These settlers sought new
and better lives for themselves and their families. Their
search for and purchase of inexpensive good land was
their driving force. Available inexpensive land attracted
many of the new settlers to the South Carolina
Backcountry. The colony's land policy was more favorable
than in Virginia and North Carolina. The male head of

a household could claim 100 acres for himself. Each member of a family, including servants, could claim an additional 50 acres. By 1750, there were about 65,000 people in South Carolina. Over the next 50 years that number would greatly increase.

In an effort to attract more settlers to South Carolina, townships were established. The townships were tracts of land set aside for settlers, similar to what had been done in New England. Many Virginia and North Carolina settlers sold their farms, packed their family and belongings into a wagon, with a cow in tow, and headed for the cheap land of South Carolina. In 1770, a man could purchase 550 acres for 200 pounds.

The settlers utilized everything they could off their farms, even the ashes from the fireplaces. Ashes were saved in a hopper where water was poured over them and allowed to drain into a container. When the lye in the container became concentrated enough to float an egg, it was combined with lard (animal fat saved from cooking) and made into soap. The lye soap was very strong and would bleach clothes or anything else it contacted, including skin.

Most of what the settlers knew about living off the land in America they learned from the Indians—how to clear the land, what crops to plant, where and when to plant, how to plant, and how and when to harvest. Many of the vegetables the Indians used—corn, squash, and potatoes—were new to the Europeans. The Indians taught the settlers how to fish and hunt. Healing Springs settlers were fortunate the Edisto Indians living near them were friendly.

One important thing settlers learned from the Indians was the use of "fat lighter," which is pine heartwood. Yellow pine heartwood was a good source of kindling for starting fires, especially when firewood was damp. Fat lighter sticks are still used today for starting fires in home fireplaces. Both Indians and settlers used fat lighter pine knots as torches to light their paths at night.

Soon, the settlers learned that a number of products could be produced from the fat lighter pine stumps for personal use and for sale. Rosin, tar, pitch, and turpentine could be made by heating the pine stumps and driving off the sap. Some of the collected sap was then sold as naval stores for use in wooden ship manufacture. Both North and South Carolina developed a large Naval Stores industry during the Colonial period. Some settlers also learned how to tap living pine trees and collect resin in metal pots hung on the side of the trees, similar to the way maple sap is collected for syrup. The collected pine resin was boiled into tar and sold. The vapors emitted from the boiling resin was distilled into turpentine, used to treat wounds and sore throats in humans and parasites in animals.

Many of the early settler homes were built out of heart yellow pine. Fence posts were made of heart yellow pine to avoid rotting and termite damage—some posts used to mark property lines still exist today. Heart pine floors of old farm homes in South Carolina are worn down halfway through two-inch thick boards. The wood was so hard and durable it was used for making troughs for watering animals, and logs were hollowed out for water pipes.

As the years went by, more and more settlers came down the Great Wagon Road. The influx of new settlers plus the very high birthrate in the late 1700s—triple the current rate—resulted in a great increase in the population. Most women bore from five to eight children, with most surviving to maturity.

One must remember that the Healing Springs community was a very remote place in the 1700s. It was about a day's ride to the Orangeburg District courthouse and there were very few travelers' rest stops, inns, and taverns along the roads. The few churches in the Backcountry served as places of social gatherings as well as houses of worship. Hector St. John de Crevecoeur, a Frenchman traveling through America in the 1750s, wrote that what distinguished the Americans from others was the widespread equality of its people, especially the rural farmers. He said they were hostile to anything smacking of aristocratic privilege. This was why the Backcountry settlers disliked most of the Lowcountry planters. Crevecoeur also stated that wealth in the Backcountry, while not distributed equally, was spread broadly. All the farmers were striving to become self-sufficient.

The Scots-Irish settlers arriving in the Backcountry were independent, undisciplined, aggressive, and family loving. Families migrated together and lived close to each other. When trouble came, they helped each other. Out of this community of settlers grew some of the strongest leaders of the Revolutionary War.

Tarlton Brown's family was one of the first to move into present-day Barnwell County. They settled on Brier's

Creek, running opposite Burton's Ferry on the Savannah River. Tarlton's father, William, was a planter in Albemarle County, Virginia. In 1769, William followed his brother Bartlet to South Carolina. According to Tarlton's memoirs, the area was very thinly inhabited and they lived in a bark tent for several weeks before constructing a log cabin. The soil was exceedingly fertile and produced abundant crops. The area was full of wild beasts, which attacked livestock and came right up to the door of the cabin. Those venturing outside after dark were usually armed. The forest was full of wild game like deer and turkey. He saw herds of fifty deer in a day's ride into the woods. The range for cattle was excellent and farmers had large herds. His family sold beef, pork, staves, and shingles. Corn was planted for consumption only, as there were few mills in the area. One interesting thing Tarlton reported was that there were many wild horses, which were caught and sold.

Before the Revolution, some of the early settlers moving into the Healing Springs area and present-day Barnwell County included the Gill family, 1765–69; the Hutto family along the Pon Pon (Edisto), 1735–37; and the Reed family near present-day Blackville, early 1700s. The Odoms were listed in the 1790 census for Orangeburg District: Benjamin Sr., Benjamin Jr., Daniel, Owen, Uriah, Isaac, Richard, and David. Elizabeth Walker, a daughter of Nathaniel Walker, married Daniel Odom. The Reeds and Clarks arrived in the mid-to-late 1700s. The head of the Clark family was Malcolm Clark, an Irish surveyor who immigrated to America in 1750 and settled near Bamberg in the Orangeburg District. King George III sent Clark to America as a surveyor for the crown. He was appointed in 1775 a Justice of the Queen for Orangeburg District, which at that time included Barnwell County. In 1776, Governor John Rutledge commissioned him a Justice of the Peace.

Once Malcolm Clark was established in America he sent for his wife, two sons, and two daughters. A family legend passed down to his ancestor Chet Matthews, owner of the Samuel and Mary Clark Reed home near Healing Springs, describes how Malcolm Clark went to the coast to meet the ship bringing his wife, son Hugh, and daughter Mary to South Carolina. When the ship arrived, it could not dock due to bad weather so Malcolm Clark, being so anxious to see his family, began rowing a boat out to the ship. As he rowed, the sea became rougher. The high waves capsized the rowboat and Clark drowned within sight of his family. Clark's friends brought the surviving family members to the Clark home where they gradually adjusted to life in the South Carolina Backcountry. Money was not a concern as Malcolm had provided well for them.

Tories killed Malcolm's son Hugh during the Revolutionary War. Daughter Mary married Samuel Reed, a prominent farmer near Healing Springs, about 1782. Within a few years, they began building their new home, which still stands today, near Healing Springs. This home, now owned by Malcolm's descendant, Chet Matthews, was completed about 1790. The beautiful two-story home has front and back porches and cedar shutters with handmade iron latches. The interior doorknobs and latches, made in England, still operate and Chet has the original keys. The floors and walls are made with wide boards. The house looks today much as it did when Samuel and Mary Clark Reed moved in.

Samuel Reed, like Malcolm Clark, was a wealthy farmer. He and Clark were Scots-Irish who immigrated to America in the mid to late 1700s from Ireland. It is likely that Malcolm Clark and Samuel Reed knew each other in Ireland or met while on the ship bringing them to South Carolina. It seems only natural that Samuel and Mary might become man and wife. They shared a common background and likely spoke English with the same strong Irish accent. Between 1783 and 1801, they had nine children. Their last child, Mary (Polly), married Austin Boylston, the author's ancestor. Polly's older brother Samuel married Elizabeth (Lizzie) Boylston, Austin's older sister.

According to family records, William (Bill) M. Odom's family was one of the first to live around Healing Springs, well before the Revolutionary War. The family included farmers, teachers, and merchants. Some of the Odom relatives included the McClendons, Reeds, Heads, Morrises, Gardners, Walkers, Peters, Keelers, Boylstons, Whittles, Cains, Williamses, and Hairs.

AMERICAN REVOLUTION

In 1763, following the end of the French and Indian War, the victorious English issued a proclamation prohibiting American settlers from moving west of the Appalachian Mountains. This move marked the beginning of increased problems between colonists and Mother England. Having been left to their own devices for so many years, the colonists resisted increased control. This limiting of freedom eventually led to war.

Each part of the country had its own unique concerns. In South Carolina, the Lowcountry planters worried about increased English taxes and trade, while the small Backcountry farmers fretted over Lowcountry control over them. Generally, people living near Healing Springs when the Revolution began had little concern about the war. They were too busy working their farms. Many believed the fight belonged to the Lowcountry planters and they did not want to be involved. Also, many of the Backcountry settlers were relative newcomers to America from Ireland and England and they still had close ties to the mother country. Backcountry settlers just wanted to be left alone.

In the colonies, there were about as many people loyal to the Crown—called Tories or Loyalists—as there were Patriots. The one thing that tended to unite communities was the threat of Indian attack by tribes bribed by the English crown. The Loyalists had the same basic political values as the Patriots and generally opposed more English taxes and controls. However, they felt these grievances were not important enough to go to war over and separate themselves from Great Britain. In 1776, twenty-five to forty percent of the Backcountry settlers were Loyalists.

The area called Backcountry began about fifty miles from the coast, in the Piedmont. The beautiful countryside was made up of low rolling hills, lush forests, numerous streams, and swampland. Major rivers like the Edisto and Savannah formed wide swamps in low-lying areas. Farmland was rich and crops plentiful. Wild game was abundant, especially in and near the swamps. Streams and rivers offered up many kinds of fish. Buffalo roamed the southeastern countryside until the mid-1700s and their paths were easy to follow.

The population in the Backcountry increased from a few settlers in 1740 to half of the total population of South Carolina by 1775. About eighty percent of all whites in South Carolina were living in the Backcountry by the time of the Revolution. This is why Backcountry men felt they deserved more representation in South Carolina government. The Backcountry men had more grievances with the South Carolina Commons House of Assembly than with the British Parliament.

As Healing Springs settlers feared, their first fighting during the American Revolution was against the Indians. The Cherokee, because of mistreatment by the colonists, sided with the British. They began attacking settlers in the Backcountry of Virginia, North Carolina, and South

Carolina. Initially, the attacks were successful because the settlers were not organized to resist.

One can only imagine what life was like on an early farm near Healing Springs when Indians attacked: About sunrise, the wife begins cooking breakfast inside the log cabin as the farmer cranks the pulley over the well outside, hauling up a bucket of fresh water. The oldest daughter milks the cow while the oldest son collects hay from the barn to feed the mules. As the farmer starts walking back toward the cabin with the bucket of water, the dogs bark wildly. Knowing they only behave this way when agitated, he runs to the lot fence to determine the problem. One quick look across the field toward the woods gives him the answer. Four Indians are emerging from the shadow of the trees through a low ground fog. The dogs' barking alerts the Indians they are detected and the element of surprise is gone. Carrying tomahawks and bows, they break into a run toward the log cabin.

The farmer shouts for his daughter and son to make haste for the house. As soon as all are safely inside, the farmer closes and barricades the door. He is not completely unprepared, as he received warning just the week before about the increasing number of Indian attacks along the Savannah River. He and his Healing Springs neighbors expected these attacks to expand to the South Edisto River. In preparation, they constructed heavy wooden shutters for all windows, with peepholes for viewing and firing weapons. The doors had similar openings. An extra supply of lead bullets and black powder was purchased.

By the time the Indians reach the farmyard, all the log cabin windows and doors are barricaded, with the farmer, his wife, daughter, son, and baby son safe inside. The farmer has two muzzle loading muskets and two pistols. He positions himself at the front door with one musket. The son, with the other musket, stands ready at the back door. The daughter and mother are stationed on each side wall with the pistols, watching from peepholes in the window shutters. On the table in the center of the cabin the supply of black powder and extra lead bullets is close at hand.

The farmer knows their only chance for survival is to make every shot count. He instructs his family not to fire unless they are certain they will hit their target. Seeing the cabin barricaded, the Indians hesitate. When they are not fired upon, they believe the farmer is too afraid to fight. They slowly approach the front door, holding tomahawks in the ready position. When they reach the door, the father thrusts the barrel of his musket through the peephole right into the chest of one of the Indians and fires. As the Indian falls, the other three run behind the barn. After awhile, the remaining three Indians separate to approach the house from different directions at once.

Deducing the attackers' plan, the farmer reloads his musket and moves to the back door. His son replaces him at the front door. The mother and daughter are warned to expect attacks from the sides of the house.

After about fifteen minutes, the Indians rush the cabin from three sides simultaneously. They do not try the front door again. Everyone inside is ready and waiting with their loaded weapons. As one of the Indians reaches the window on the north side of the house where the mother is positioned he begins pulling at the shutters. At that, the mother thrusts her pistol through the peephole and fires it directly at the Indian's shoulder. The bleeding Indian yelps, then runs toward the woods.

At the same time the Indians at the back door and on the south side of the house are attacking. The brave at the back door learned his lesson well and stands to the side of the door and kicking it and striking the latch with his tomahawk. The father has no clear shot, so he waits and watches. Having hunted turkeys on the high ground along the river, he knows the importance of patience. Each time the Indian strikes the door latch with his tomahawk he exposes the side of his head. The next time he strikes, the farmer shoots, grazing the Indian's scalp. The farmer hears the brave holler, then sees him running away.

About the time the farmer fires, he hears one of the pistols fire. After the Indian at the back door runs, he rushes to the side of the cabin. There, his daughter stands, holding a smoking pistol. Looking through the peephole, he sees a dead Indian lying on the ground.

The attack lasts only a few minutes, but it feels like hours. Of the four Indians attacking the cabin, two are dead and two wounded. The last the farmer sees of Indians that day is the two wounded heading into the woods, one holding his head and the other his shoulder. The two would not tarry long enough on this occasion to get Healing Springs water to treat their injuries.

Once the farmer sees the way is clear, he opens the

front door and checks to be sure the two fallen Indians are dead. Both lay where they were shot, one at the front door and one at the side window. The family thanks God for sparing their lives and their home. After a while, the farmer and his son get their shovels and dig a grave by the edge of the woods. Both Indians are placed in the same grave and a large stone is set up as a marker. The farmer decides to keep the two dead Indians' tomahawks as a reminder of the attack and hangs them on a peg over the fireplace. There they would hang for the remainder of the farmer's life, then pass on to the farmer's son and his son's sons.

This attack was similar to many by Indians on South Carolina Backcountry settlers before and during the Revolutionary War. Settlers began to organize retaliatory expeditions. By the end of 1777 these expeditions had burned the majority of Cherokee towns and forced the Indians to sign treaties ceding most of the South Carolina land to the colony. The Indians were forced away from their homeland of thousands of years and there were no more Indian attacks (because there were no more Indians).

In 1775, Tory militia units in the Backcountry began attacking Patriot troops. After savage fighting, the Tories were defeated. The conflict shifted to the coast, where a British invasion force was bested at Sullivan's Island. Following these fights, things calmed down for a while.

Healing Springs settlers had little contact with Tories or the British troops in the first few years of the Revolutionary War. Then in 1778, the British formulated a new strategy and focused their attention on the South where they believed they would have more local support. Also, France and Spain were fighting Britain and the British needed southern seaports to protect their West Indies holdings. A British force of 3,500 troops took Savannah, Georgia, in 1778. With the aid of the many Loyalist militiamen in the South, the British planned to capture all key seaports.

On May 12, 1780, Gen. Henry Clinton captured Charles Town, South Carolina, with 9,000 British troops. After Charleston fell, the British, with the help of the large number of Upcountry Loyalists, expected to control all of South Carolina. There were thousands of Loyalists enlisted in Royal militia units in the Carolinas. Most of these were recent Scots-Irish and Scotch immigrants. However, the Cherokee Indian attacks had caused many of the Loyalists to switch sides. The remaining Loyalists engaged in bloody fights with the Patriots—some of the bloodiest fighting of the entire war. In 1782 there was a continuous cycle of revenge, retribution, and retaliation. The war in South Carolina became a personal conflict.

Thomas Sumter and Andrew Pickens, two of South Carolina's foremost generals, took up arms only after Tories raided their plantations in 1780. Another South Carolinian, Tory William Cunningham, nicknamed Bloody Bill, walked sixty miles to find and kill a Patriot officer who had his brother whipped to death. Then he became a Loyalist guerrilla, raiding Patriots' homes until the end of the war. The British and Tories used fear and brutality in the South Carolina Backcountry to coerce citizens. Such tactics did not work and caused more settlers to join the Patriot ranks. A number of partisan bands were formed under the leadership of Thomas Sumter ("Gamecock"), Francis Marion ("Swamp Fox"), and others. A great civil war resulted, with sons and fathers fighting each other, neighbors fighting neighbors, and friends fighting former friends. One Patriot is reported to have claimed that the only thing a man could trust was his rifle.

Once the South Carolina Backcountry men decided to fight the British for independence, the Revolutionary War began to turn in favor of the Patriots. The men of the Backcountry played a major role in winning the American Revolution. Some of the major decisive battles were fought in South Carolina's Backcountry, including Kings Mountain and Cowpens.

On April 9, 1780, a British fleet of fourteen ships appeared off the Charleston coast. Another British invasion force landed on John's Island. The five thousand colonial troops in Charleston were surrounded and on May 12, 1780, the city surrendered. With this, there was no longer a colonial army to oppose the British in the South. The British then occupied a number of Backcountry towns, including Rocky Mount, Hanging Rock, Ninety Six, Camden, and Cheraw. When British general Clinton ordered all citizens to pledge allegiance to the king, many remaining Backcountry Loyalists turned against the British. British Legion commander Banastre Tarleton turned many American settlers against the British when his men killed unarmed Patriots. One Patriot officer survived over twenty stab wounds. The Backcountry men responded like hornets in a disturbed nest, attacking the British outposts repeatedly.

There remained at this point very few Loyalists around Healing Springs. Because they formed such a small minority, they kept quiet. In August 1780, British general Cornwallis, who had relieved Clinton, defeated Gen. Horatio Gates at Camden, South Carolina. The war was moving inland to the Backcountry and by this time fighting was about seventy-five miles away from Healing Springs. Gates was replaced by Patriot general Nathanael Greene, who continued to lose battles but ultimately won the campaign in South Carolina and North Carolina, since he protected the Patriot militia. Greene caused the British supply lines to be extended and inflicted heavy casualties on the British. Finally, Cornwallis was forced to leave the Carolinas for Virginia.

Many Healing Springs natives fought with the local Whig militia and likely participated in the battles of King's Mountain and Cowpens in South Carolina and Guilford Courthouse in North Carolina. Some Healing Springs settlers likely continued with General Greene to Yorktown and participated in the final defeat of the British.

Tarlton Brown described in his Revolutionary War memoirs what life was like during the conflict in what is now Barnwell County. When the war broke out in 1775, Brown was drafted and sent to Pocotaligo under General Bull's command. After about seven weeks he was discharged and returned home just in time for another draft. This time he was not drafted, but was paid by William Bryant to serve for him during the first siege of Savannah.

He served under the command of Captain Moore and traveled by boat for three days to Savannah. Brown was there about seven weeks under enemy fire and was struck once by a spent ball.

In 1776, Brown enlisted in the regular service in Beaufort District in Capt. William Harden's company of about eighty-five soldiers. In July 1777 he accompanied Capt. John Mumford on an expedition to Georgia where they attacked the British in a barricaded house. After the captain and others were wounded, the group returned to South Carolina.

Following the capture of Charles Town by British general Henry Clinton, Captain Mumford and his men attempted to join the Continental troops when they were attacked at Morris Ford on the Salkehatchie River by Old Ben John and his gang of Tories. Mumford was killed and buried under a large pine tree near where he fell. Soon after this skirmish, Brown accompanied fifty horsemen under the command of Colonel Thompson and Major Bourguoin in attacking Tories under Captain Mott. They surprised the Tories and captured all of them.

Tarlton Brown, Joshua Inman, and John Green, formed a company of Ranger horsemen at Cracker's Neck, South Carolina. From there the company roamed the area attacking British and Tories. Once while traveling near his home, Brown stopped for a visit. About midnight barking dogs awakened him, just before a group of Tories knocked at the door. The men claimed they were friends from Sister's Ferry and General Lincoln's army and needed a place to stay for the night. When Brown told them there was no room, they began to whisper among themselves. Finally, they asked for a torch so they could build a camp-fire at Brier's Creek. Brown opened the door, handed them a torch, and quickly closed the door. Looking through a crack above the door, he recognized the illuminated faces of the men as Tories. The men then asked for water. When directed to the well in the yard, they began shouting threats. They hammered on the door with their fists, then shot through a crack between the logs four or five times, killing Brown's little brother. The Brown family grabbed their weapons and the Tories retreated, firing at the log cabin from a safe distance before they departed.

According to Tarlton Brown, the entire countryside seemed to be in complete subjugation to the British and the Tories. He, like other Backcountry Patriots, hated the Tories. He wrote, "They who had grown up side by side, and hand in hand, together, father and son, and brother, were arrayed in mortal and ferocious strife against each other."

During a scouting trip on the Edisto River, Tory captain James Roberts and his men captured and killed many Patriots, always escaping capture themselves. Tarlton Brown volunteered to pursue them with Captain Vince. The Patriots caught up with the Tories at "the Ford of the Edisto" and killed five or six of them. Then the Patriot troop went to Captain Salley's "Cowpens" a few miles distance. The road leading to Salley's Cowpens was from the southwest toward John's Town and about a mile west of present-day Salley, South Carolina. Brown described an ambush, likely of the South Edisto River ford near present-day Guinyard's Bridge. According to Brown, when Tory captain Roberts rode to a mill nearby, he was fired upon and wounded in an ambush. The author's great-great grandfather, John Corbitt, owned this mill and pond. Later, in the war, the Patriots under Captains Salley and William Butler would meet and defeat a band of Tories near this mill at the battle of Little Cowpens.

Tarlton Brown described how, on one occasion, he and his companion, John Cave, observed a company of about 150 mounted Tories under the command of Chaney and Williams head toward Captain Vince's station on the Savannah River. Brown and Cave rode rapidly to warn the fort, which had only twenty-five defenders. Hearing of the large force approaching, the Patriots evacuated. Finding the fort empty, the Tories continued toward their headquarters on the Edisto. At Lower Three Runs Creek, they stopped at the Collins house and killed the eighty-five-year-old Mr. Collins.

Surrounded by British troops and Tories near the Savannah River, Tarlton Brown and his brother Bartlet rode toward Virginia (likely what is now western North Carolina) with a small group of refugees. It was during this same bloody period that McGeart and his company of Tories crossed the Savannah River from Georgia into present-day Barnwell County at Summerlin's Ferry (later called Stone's Ferry) where they killed every man not swearing allegiance to the King. They killed seventeen people near Brown's home including his father, Henry Best, and a man named Moore. John Cave was left for dead but recovered. Brown's house was burned and everything of value destroyed.

Brown also fought with Gen. Francis Marion in the swamps and at Monk's Corner. He later left Marion and joined a detachment of eighty men under Colonels Harden and Baker and Maj. John Cooper. The detachment's route was by "the Four Holes" and across the Edisto at Givan's Ferry. Coming upon a group of Tories under Captain Barton, the Patriots attacked and killed most of them.

Brown participated in skirmishes around Augusta, Georgia, and attacked Tory boats on the Savannah River and at Silver Bluff. He fought in the siege of Augusta in April 1781. Soon after, he contracted smallpox and was sent home for forty days. He returned to duty, serving under Major Cooper at Beech Island until the end of the war in 1782.

Tarlton Brown returned to his home in present-day Barnwell County and found the Tories and British had destroyed everything he owned. Soon after his return, his mother died. Despite the British surrender, some Tories continued their plundering and killing. Brown and others chased the Tories all the way to Tennessee, capturing and returning them to South Carolina.

Brown finally settled down between the Sand Hill and Cedar Branches of Lower Three Runs Creek in Barnwell District. There he built mills. In later life, he moved to Boiling Springs.

The Backcountry of South Carolina was a bloody battleground during the American Revolution. During the first four years of the war (1775-1779), the area saw few skirmishes. Beginning in 1779, that changed. To 1782 more than 125 battles were fought across the state. The most famous battles in the Backcountry were Camden, King's Mountain, and Cowpens. It is interesting to note that the first Revolutionary War action in South Carolina occurred at the Backcountry's Fort Charlotte near Mount Carmel, thirty miles southwest of Ninety-Six. This fort guarded a ford over the Savannah River used by Creek Indians to raid the settlers. In June 1775, Maj. James Mayson, a Patriot from Ninety-Six, was ordered to capture the fort, which he did. During this time one of the attackers, Kirkland, changed sides and almost started a civil war.

On June 28, 1776, British warships attacked Fort Moultrie on Sullivan's Island at Charles Town Harbor. The sand and palmetto log fort held and the British withdrew. The next time the British returned to Charleston they approached the city by land. Before reaching Charleston, the British fought a number of skirmishes including those near the Salkehatchie River on March 18, 1780, and the Edisto River on March 23, where Col. Banastre Tarleton struck a party of Patriots, killing ten and capturing four. This battle was known as the Pon Pon (Edisto) battle.

The British, under the command of Sir Henry Clinton, opened fire on Charleston on April 11, 1780. On May 11, the city, with 5,600 soldiers, 1,000 sailors, and 400 artillery pieces, surrendered.

The 3rd Virginia Regiment of Continentals, about 350 men, commanded by Col. Abraham Buford, was the last remaining Continental force in South Carolina after the fall of Charleston. Clinton sent Cornwallis with 2,500 infantry and Tarleton's cavalry to attack Buford. Tarleton caught Buford about seven miles from present-day Lancaster. The British cavalry killed 113 Patriot officers and men. This battle of the Waxhaws gave Tarleton an unenviable reputation—for brutality and refusing to give quarter to those surrendering. "Tarleton's Quarter" became an American battle cry synonymous with "take no prisoners."

One of the bloodiest and costliest Patriot defeats of the Revolution occurred at Camden, South Carolina, on August 16, 1780. The British seemed to have complete control of the state. However, Generals Marion and Pickens continued to harass the British. Col. William Harden fought with Marion for a while before operating in the Lowcountry between Savannah and Charleston. Tarlton Brown fought with Harden.

Silver Bluff on the Savannah River, about 30 miles from Healing Springs was the site of a number of Revolutionary War skirmishes. On May 21, 1781, British troops were at Fort Galphin on the South Carolina side of the river at Silver Bluff. This fort consisted of trader George Galphin's house surrounded by a stockade fence. The Aiken County Historical Commision moved one of Galphin's houses in the early 1960s from the Savannah River Site. Not long after being moved it burned.

The British called Galphin's fort Fort Drednough. This fort became very important in May 1781 since supplies for the Indians allied with the British were sent there for distribution. For years the British had given presents

73

to the Indians on an annual basis to retain their loyalty. This time the shipment contained not only presents but also ordinance and quartermaster stores. Once the Patriots learned of the shipment, they set out to capture the flotilla. Col. Elijah Clarke of Georgia was placed in command of the company. Clarke attacked the boats but was unable to prevent them from reaching Fort Galphin. At the fort, the British were surrounded and they could expect no help from Augusta, since Patriot general Andrew Pickens had cut off the city. Col. Henry Lee aided Pickens with some of Gen. Thomas Sumter's troops. Cavalry major John Rudolph was sent with some Lee's cavalry to help capture the fort at Silver Bluff.

Major Rudolph used a small decoy force to lure the British outside the fort. Once the British were in the open, Rudolph charged them, rushing through the open gate. Four redcoats were killed and 126 captured, including 70 regulars. Only one Patriot died, apparently from heat exhaustion, and 10 were wounded. The supplies captured at Fort Galphin helped the Patriots take Augusta on June 5, 1781.

Life around Healing Springs was rough before and during the Revolution. The entire South Carolina Backcountry had been in turmoil for over twenty years. Most settlers worked hard from dawn to dusk. Besides laboring on their farms, they often had to fight Indians and outlaws. Then the war began and they fought the Tories and the British. As a result of their hard life, the early settlers became an independent, tough, self-reliant people, firm in their beliefs about religion and government. They were not about to let anyone push them around. Despite the fact that many of the Backcountry settlers wanted to remain neutral, they ended up fighting those who attacked, whether they were redcoat, Loyalist, or Indian. Life in the Backcountry produced excellent guerrilla fighters, as the British found out the hard way.

Atrocities were committed on both sides in the war. This was vividly portrayed in the movie *The Patriot*. One of the most notorious villains was Major "Bloody Bill" Cunningham, a Tory who led many raids into the Backcountry. Cunningham attacked a party of thirty Patriots under Captain Turner in present-day Lexington County. Seeing Cunningham's superior force, Turner offered to surrender. Cunningham refused to accept since it would free James Butler, Jr., who had killed one of Cunningham's men. Butler's father offered to give his life for his son, but Cunningham refused that offer as well. When the fight began, young Butler was mortally wounded. Following the surrender, Cunningham killed Captain Turner, the senior Butler, and the other Patriots— except the two who escaped to tell the story.

One important Revolutionary War skirmish in present-day Barnwell County was the battle of Slaughter Field, which occurred near Windy Hill Creek. Windy Hill runs northeast behind Healing Springs, across present-day Highway 3, toward South Edisto River. The battle occurred about one mile northwest of the intersection of county roads S-6-87 (Jones Bridge Road) and S-6-32 (Healing Springs Road).

In August 1781, Lt. Col. Banastre Tarleton ("The

Butcher") sent a company of 150 Tories to harass the Patriots at Ninety-Six. The Tories were commanded by "Bloody Bill" Cunningham. Col. Hezekiah Williams's troops accompanied him. The Tories were proceeding along the Indian trail on the south side of South Edisto River when they encountered a group of Patriots camped on Windy Hill Creek near Healing Springs. There was a bloody fight during which all the Patriots were killed.

An Indian girl, believed to be with the group of Patriots, escaped and traveled by foot to Ninety-Six ahead of the Tories to warn them of the attack. All Patriots killed at Slaughter Field, likely including some from the Healing Springs community, lay on the field for three days before relatives could bury them.

According to local history, four redcoats with Cunningham at the battle of Slaughter Field were wounded and left at Healing Springs to die. Two Tories were left to take care of the wounded until they died and were then to return to Charles Town. Six months later, the two men caring for the dying redcoats arrived in Charles Town accompanied by the four wounded redcoats. It appears the water of Healing Springs heals enemies as well as friends. News of the recovery of the wounded soldiers and the waters of Healing Springs spread throughout South Carolina. The legend of Healing Springs continued to grow.

Healing Springs
by *Alice Cabaniss*

Mark this place water bubbling from the ground
Where sapling lighten in April sun is all you see
Unless you know the legend of the flowing spring.
See some blood
Here, the passing Indian believed, clear, magic waters rose,
Obeying some compassioned stirring of gods.
Knowing where to find these soothing streams.
Cut the natives' arrow flight the shorter.
Gave the shealth more daring knotted muscles in his arm
Shivering before the British musket, did he trade
His captured life for such a secret, lead the soldiers
To the spring where wounds might wash and mend?
Two hundred years of echoes reinforce the story.
Shadows of the resurrected redcoats
Brought the farmer with his bucket to the ever-flowing stream.
Mark this place.
Its air saturate with sounds
Of dying and living, with ancient blood
Upon the logs and silent butterflies between.

Following their victory at Camden on August 16, 1780, the British had moved farther into the Backcountry. They were attacked by Patriots and defeated at Kings Mountain on October 7. On January 17, 1781, the Patriots, under command of Brig. Gen. Daniel Morgan, defeated the British regulars at Cowpens. General Cornwallis pursued Morgan into North Carolina. Maj. Gen. Nathanael Greene, who had been appointed commander of the Patriot Army in the South, joined Morgan in fighting Cornwallis at Guilford Courthouse near present-day Greensboro on March 15, 1781. Cornwallis pushed the Patriots back, but because of his heavy losses, decided it was best to retreat to Wilmington. From there, he marched to Virginia, surrendering at Yorktown on October 19, 1781. Thus, it can be seen that the independence of the American colonies was greatly determined by the final battles won by the Backcountry men of the Carolinas.

In many respects the Patriot partisan bands were as bad as the Tories. Thomas Sumter's band searched for booty everywhere they went. Sumter had offered payment of one slave to any private signing up for ten months. A major received three slaves for a year's enlistment. During the Revolutionary War, about twenty five percent of South Carolina's slaves disappeared. One of the slaves Thomas Sumter captured belonged to William Bennett Boylston's daughter-in-law, Alice Cloud, who would later settle at Healing Springs. Alice was living in Winnsboro, South Carolina, at the time Sumter's troops came through on their way to North Carolina. The slave woman captured was her personal servant, given to her by her father in his will. The slave had raised Alice from a small child. She continued to take care of her mistress until one of Sumter's officers snatched her while marching through the streets of Winnsboro. William Boylston and his son George, upon learning the former slave was taken to North Carolina, brought suit against her captor in the Salisbury court. Since the statue of limitations had expired, he lost his suit. Later William's wife and son, George, asked the South Carolina House of Representatives to authorize payment for the stolen slave. Their request was denied since the statue of limitations for reimbursement for war claims had expired in the state.

There was an estimated 1,000 Americans killed in action throughout the colonies in 1780. Sixty-six percent of these died in South Carolina, most of them in the Backcountry. During the last two years of the Revolutionary War 1,089 Patriots died in South Carolina. This represented eighteen percent of all American deaths in the entire Revolutionary War. For South Carolina, the war would not end until December 14, 1782, when the British left Charles Town with 4,200 Loyalists.

Healing Springs natives were well represented in the Patriot forces during the Revolution, especially the Walker family. Nathaniel Walker, Sr., and four of his sons fought: Capt. Nathaniel Walker, Jr. (1744-1801); Capt. William Walker (1757-1807); Lt. George Walker (1759-1800); and Pvt. John Walker (1755-?).

POST REVOLUTION

The 1790 United States census documented about four million people living in the nation, mostly along the Atlantic coast. A mere 100,000 hardy souls lived west of the Allegheny Mountains. Roads and methods of communication were still poor. Two stagecoaches and twelve horses carried all passenger land traffic between New York City and Boston. It took about a month for news of the Declaration of Independence to travel from Philadelphia to Charles Town.

One must remember that 500 years ago, there were no European settlers in the United States, and 300 years ago there were only a few settlements along the Atlantic coast. The United States was in its infancy a mere 225 years ago.

Soon after the end of the Revolutionary War and the slackening of hostilities in the South Carolina Backcountry, there was a great influx of new settlers to Winton (later, Barnwell) County. Some of the many new families in the 1700s included those of Lewis Malone Ayer, Jr., a courier for Gen. Francis Marion, about 1793; the James Arthur Bates family, about 1790; the Carroll family; the Thomas Gill family; the John Hair family, about 1790; the Isaac Hutto family, about 1737; the Thomas O'Bannon family, about 1770; and the William Reed family, about 1790. There were 326 taxable persons in Winton County in 1784. Winton County was part of

Orangeburg District in 1785. Orangeburg District had four courthouses (counties): Orangeburg, Lexington, Lewisburg, and Winton.

After six years as Winton, the county became known as Barnwell in 1800. It included most of present-day Aiken, Bamberg, Barnwell, and Allendale Counties. At that time the entire area was mostly forest with a few scattered villages, including Windsor, Aiken, Barnwell, Boiling Springs, and Healing Springs. However, the word was spreading throughout South Carolina and beyond about the rich, fertile land between the South Edisto and Savannah Rivers. Thus, many new settlers began moving into the area.

Typical of the families moving into the Healing Springs area of Winton County was the Boylston family. John Boylston of Leeds, County Essex, England; his wife Lidia Elliot; and their son Thomas sailed to Boston in 1647 on the ship *Defense*. Thomas later married Elizabeth Bennett of Virginia. Thomas and Elizabeth's son William married Mary Thornton of Virginia, a neighbor of George Washington. William and Mary's son Thomas married Mahulda Box. Their son William Bennett married Joanna Austin of Fredericksburg, Virginia. William and Joanna had one child, George.

In the early 1780s, William, Joanna, and their son George, along with George's wife Alice Hardin Cloud moved from Virginia to Winnsboro, South Carolina, with some of the Cloud family. They were seeking new opportunities and more land. William had fought in the Revolutionary War in Virginia along with his brothers and uncles.

About 1790, the Boylstons purchased a few hundred acres bordering the South Edisto River, north of Healing Springs in Winton County. Much of the land was covered with forest. However, there was an old Indian and trader trail leading to a natural landing on the river. The move from Winnsboro to Healing Springs was about seventy-five miles over poor roads through Orangeburg District and across the South Edisto River at what would become Holman's Bridge, east of where the Boylston home would be located. As other settlers of their day, the family traveled by horse and wagon, bringing all their belongings with them. They spent one night in Orangeburg before continuing their trip. There were a number of travelers' rest stops across the state at that time where travelers could obtain lodging and meals.

During these early days of Winton (Barnwell) County, there were few bridges. Small streams were crossed at fords, and ferries were used for large streams and rivers. The ferries were usually flat-bottom boats pulled by large ropes stretched across the river. Most ferries would hold only one wagon and the mules pulling it.

This trip to the Healing Springs community was the second for William and George Boylston. About three months earlier they had come to the area and built a log cabin on their new property. They lived in a tent while constructing the cabin on the high ground a few hundred yards south of the South Edisto River landing, later Boylston Landing. All the trees needed for constructing the cabin came from their property. Saws and axes were used to bring down the trees. Once felled, the trunks were cleared and the logs pulled to the cabin site by mules. After the cabin walls were complete, a wood shingle roof was installed.

The log cabin had one main room that served as kitchen, dining room, and sitting area. There were two bedrooms on one end. Local stones were brought in by wagon to build a large chimney at the end of the cabin opposite the bedrooms. A porch was added to the front of the cabin. William and George built the log cabin in a location where it would later serve as the kitchen for a larger permanent house.

Next, they built a shed for the mules and cows and set up a lot to keep them in at night. A well would be dug later. In the meantime, water would be hauled from the river and nearby springs.

As the Boylston family approached their new home on South Edisto River, they were excited about settling down at a permanent location. They arrived the first day near sundown and had time only to put the mules in the lot and unload what they needed for the first night.

While William took care of the mules, George built a fire in the fireplace and hauled a bucket of water from the river. Soon Joanna and Alice were brewing coffee and cooking salt-cured ham, grits, and biscuits. Of course, there was a jug of sugar cane syrup for the biscuits. It was the first of many meals the Boylstons would enjoy in the small log cabin before building the big house by the large oak trees not far away.

William, an experienced carpenter, taught George carpentry skills. Together they built all the family needed for their cabin: cabinets, shelves, beds, tables, and benches. At the same time they completed a small barn, a smokehouse, and chicken pens. Although there were not many people living nearby, the few neighbors welcomed the new family to the community, bringing food and offering assistance. The Walkers were the first to come and they invited the newcomers to the local Edisto Baptist Church. Within a few months, the Boylston family had established its homestead. Each summer they cleared more land and planted more crops.

While the lives of new settlers were improving, the lives of native Americans were deteriorating. The desire of settlers for more land drove the Indians away, forcing them to move west. Some fled to the mountains and others to the swamps along South Edisto River. A few remained on the edge of the swamp for the next thirty-five years living in huts and blending into the community.

Five years after Ben Franklin and John Adams signed the Treaty of Paris on September 3, 1783, officially ending the Revolutionary War, farmers around Healing Springs were just emerging from the destruction of the war. John Adams, who became the second president of the United States, was William Boylston's cousin. Susanna Boylston was John Adams's mother. After signing the treaty, Adams affixed his ring seal in wax on the document. This seal belonged to the Boylstons, his mother's family. Today the National Archives in Washington, DC, is home to the original treaty with the Boylston family seal for all to see.

Settlers flooded into the Backcountry when the war was over. Generally, living in the area was safe. However, there were still incidents of outlaws attacking travelers and homesteaders. More pressure was placed on state government to provide better law enforcement and courts. The general lack of money in South Carolina caused problems. Many debtors lost their property and were angry and frightened. As in the past, they took the law into their own hands. When notices of sales were posted, there was a violent response. Settlers ripped down the notices and set the courthouse afire. Soon more Backcountry courts were established. To help ease the problem of travel, in 1786 the state capital was relocated from Charles Town to Columbia.

There was general concern in the Backcountry about the ratification of the United States Constitution. Settlers did not want a stronger federal government, which they believed would not be responsive to their needs. They had experienced similar lack of response by the colonial government in Charles Town.

Gradually, farmers around Healing Springs recovered from the ravages of war and began a significant period of improvement. They produced staple crops for worldwide markets, increasing their prosperity. The war had ended the indigo trade with England's textile mills and South Carolina farmers began searching for new sources of revenue. While Lowcountry plantations shifted to rice, the Backcountry shifted to cotton. Short staple cotton, called upland or green seed cotton, began to transform South Carolina and the southeastern United States. The main difficulty with the short staple cotton was the manual separatation of the seed from the fiber. The labor force was not large enough to handle the large quantities of cotton. All that changed in 1793 when Eli Whitney, on a visit to a Savannah plantation, developed the idea for the cotton gin. Gins were manufactured and cotton production increased significantly. Community gins were established near Healing Springs where owners were paid in seed or part of the cotton.

The cotton boom lasted from 1793 until 1819. During this boom there was an increased need for labor to plow, plant, hoe, and pick but not enough laborers to meet the need. In the Lowcountry, labor needs in the rice fields were met through the use of slaves. Larger farmers in the Backcountry began to buy more slaves to work in the cotton fields in the early 1800s. Use of slaves continued to increase. In 1820, thirty to forty-nine percent of Barnwell County's population was black.

Cotton sold for 30.8 cents per pound in 1818. It is likely it sold for more in the late 1790s. Many settlers, including those around Healing Springs, who grew cotton during that period significantly increased their wealth. Another factor in the increase of cotton production was the movement of many South Carolinians to other southern states where there was cheap land. Some large families around Healing Springs had their older sons move to Georgia, Alabama, Mississippi, and Texas to start new cotton farms. Between 1820 and 1860 about 200,000 South Carolinians moved to other states—50,000 to Georgia, 45,000 to Alabama, and 20,000 to Mississippi.

In clearing their lands for crops, Healing Springs farmers had plenty of timber for sale. During the late 1700s and early 1800s river levels were higher and the flow much stronger. Logs were tied together and snaked downstream. Those transporting logs rode rafts covered with straw and dirt. At meal time, they would build fires on the rafts and cook their meals. Each night they tied up their logs and raft at a landing.

COLONIAL RELIGION

Religion was an important part of colonial life. Among the Christians leaving Europe for America in the early 1600s were the Baptists and their early leader, John Smyth, a clergyman in the Church of England. About 1607 Smyth traveled with other English exiles to the Netherlands, later returning to England. This same group was among the pilgrims sailing to America in 1620. Before leaving the Netherlands, Smyth and thirty-six other exiles formed a Baptist church.

In the 1630s the Puritan outlook in England was dark. King Charles had dissolved Parliament in 1629 and inaugurated a period of personal rule, which lasted until 1640. Nonconforming Puritans fell into displeasure and no longer had a voice in government. Then England suffered a severe textile industry depression. These adverse conditions forced the Puritans to emigrate. Thus began the Great Migration to America between 1630 and 1643. John Winthrop led seventeen ships and 2,000 settlers to Massachusetts in March 1630. During the first winter in New England, about 200 died; the following spring 200 returned to England.

In 1639 Roger Williams established a Baptist church in Providence, Rhode Island. From that point forward there was rapid growth in the Baptist Church in America. By 1800 the Baptists made up the largest Protestant group in the New World. The early churches, such as the one at

Healing Springs, served as religious centers, town halls, and social centers. Church officers, like Nathaniel Walker, often performed public services now handled by government agencies. Churches kept important records of marriages, births, deaths, and baptisms.

More than half the books written by colonial writers prior to 1700 concerned religion. Most settlers at that time were English—Anglican in the South and Puritan in New England. Of all the religious sects in America, the Baptist Church, perhaps more than any other denomination, had less connection with the old country.

The organized Baptist movement in colonial South Carolina began in 1699 with Englishman William Screven. Screven had agitated the people of Maine during his initial stop in North America with his "blasphemous" speeches about baptism by immersion. The old Baptist preacher and a small group of his followers decided to move to the South. They settled in the "Somerton" area, about forty miles upriver from Charles Town. This location was likely chosen because of prior settlements of Baptists along the Ashley, Cooper, and Stono Rivers. In late 1699 Screven moved his group of Baptists to Charles Town where they erected a church downtown, now 62 Church Street. The First Baptist Church of Charles Town is still located at that site.

The Screven Charles Town Baptist Church reflected a Calvinistic view of the scriptures. The Anglicans looked on the Baptists with amusement, and sometimes alarm, because of their baptism by immersion rather than sprinkling. By 1710 about ten percent of South Carolina's population was Baptist, with membership in the Backcountry increasing. By 1772 half of all South Carolina Baptists lived in the Backcountry. This number increased to about seventy percent by 1800.

Nathaniel Walker, likely of Irish descent, was an Anglican and the first settler in the Healing Springs area. He had served as a preacher before settling in Healing Springs and desired to establish a church there. Walker visited the Charles Town Anglican Diocese and requested they send a clergyman to the Healing Springs area so a church could be established there. He returned home believing the Anglicans would respond positively to his request. Hearing nothing after six months, Walker took matters into his own hands. If the Anglican Church would not assist him, he decided, he would start his own church and pastor the congregation himself. Walker's first congregation, which met in a log cabin near Reeves Creek, included members of many different faiths. Eventually, because of the predominance of Baptists, the church became a Baptist church. Later, another log cabin church was built on Windy Hill Creek, not far from Healing Springs. Founded in 1772, it was known as Edisto Church. A new church was constructed near Healing Springs years later and remains today in that location. Over time, three separate church buildings stood on the site. In 1804 the congregation was incorporated as "The Baptist Church in Christ of the Healing Springs in the Barnwell District." The existing church sanctuary, which stands about 100 yards north of the springs, was built in 1853 with slave labor.

During the time Nathaniel Walker was establishing

the Edisto Church, a great religious awakening swept through the colonies. This occurred in part because of the diphtheria epidemic of 1737–38. This highly contagious and deadly throat disease spread like wildfire, killing about ten percent of all children under age sixteen. The tragedy quickened the religious fervor.

There were many preachers of all faiths traveling the countryside spreading the Word of God and meeting with families and communities. They spoke of the emptiness of material things, the corruption of human nature, the fury of divine wrath, and the need for immediate repentance. Such preaching appealed to the Backcountry settlers who faced numerous hardships and death. The religious awakening split the Protestant church in America. Many churches were established during this period, particularly Baptist churches. One of these was the Edisto Church, which would later become the Healing Springs Baptist Church.

Baptist churches located in Barnwell District originally belonged to the Charles Town Association, organized in 1751. In 1803 the churches became part of the new Savannah River Association. In 1821 the first South Carolina Baptist Convention was organized.

The early Baptist associations did not accept all new churches applying for membership. This was due in part to the way the local Healing Springs Baptists, and Baptists in general, practiced their religion. Members believed it was the business of the church to see that all members lived their lives as nearly as possible in sync with God's Holy Word. They felt that church business and their personal lives should conform as much as possible to instructions laid out in the Bible. Although this may seem overly strict today, at that time religious leaders took every word of their covenant with God and their church solemnly and were not tolerant of those who thought and acted differently.

Some of the new churches applying for membership were turned down because of unfavorable reports from visiting pastors. Reports were critical, for example, of one widow marrying his late wife's sister and another member having more than one wife, simultaneously. Not only were some churches turned down, some were thrown out and individual members dismissed. The Healing Springs Baptist Church was no different from the others. Church records show many cases where members were disciplined about various religious matters.

A good example of how the Healing Springs Church felt appears in the church records in the covenant the church adopted in 1847 and was signed by all church members in 1858. Rule 7 states, "If any member shall fail to attend three conferences in secession, the cause shall be inquired into, and if found to be willful neglect, the said member shall be dealt with accordingly." Rule 8 states, "It is inconsistent with Christianity and the Teachings of the Sacred Scriptures, thus members of the church are prohibited from dancing, playing cards, using dice and billiard playing and all like amusements." This rule, No. 8, was added in 1866. Before that time, it never occurred to religious leaders a Christian would be involved in any of these things. Possibly, this problem began with members who served in the Confederate Army, returning to their homes and churches after the war with bad habits.

Church members could be charged and brought before the monthly church conference or business meeting about their unChristian conduct. Before a member could be charged, however, the matter had to be thoroughly investigated by a committee of designated church members. The church members serving on the committee would visit the member and confront him or her with the charge. The person charged was given the opportunity to explain the circumstances surrounding his or her transgression. Sometimes the member confessed and asked for forgiveness. Uusually the individual would ask the church "to wait on" him or her for a change of heart before being excluded. Until the early 1900s, women were excluded from church conferences and business meetings. They were present only when charged with adultery, drunkenness, holding of grudges, and gossip.

Now, as in the early days of settlement, the church remains the very heart and soul of the Healing Springs community.

LIFE ON THE FARM

Settled into their log cabin, George and Alice Boylston began planning their new home. Their first child, William, was born just before they left Winnsboro for Healing Springs. In 1792, they had a daughter, Annie, who died young. Then, beginning in 1794, almost yearly, they added to their family: Jane, 1794; George Jr., 1795; Cynthia, 1796; Elizabeth, 1797; Joseph, 1799; Jason, 1801; and Austin, 1802. This large number of children was typical of South Carolina farm families in the late 1700s and early 1800s. It is easy to see why large farm houses were needed. Even with four children to a room, multiple bedrooms were needed. Also, large families meant need for large amounts of food and clothing.

Healing Springs farmers worked hard. Most grew corn, beans, pumpkins, and other vegetables. They raised pigs, chickens, and cattle, which were allowed to roam freely. Early settlers learned from the Indians where to find salt and how to cook wild game like turkeys. Hams were smoked in smokehouses and fish were salted and dried. Corn was a staple and eaten in many forms, usually in cornbread. Cornmeal was mixed with milk, eggs, salt, and animal fat, then fried or baked on a griddle or in a Dutch oven. Sometimes cornbread was baked by placing it in the hot ashes of the fireplace. Such cornbread was called ashcake, hoecake, johnnycake, or corn pone. A favorite way to use corn was to grind it into grits and boil it in water. (This is still a favorite dish down South and is now being introduced up North.) Corn was harvested about mid-July. It was roasted in the shuck or shucked and boiled. To meet the growing need of farmers for more grits, local streams around Healing Springs were dammed and grist mills built. Other mills specialized in grinding wheat into flour. As more flour mills were built, farmers began to use more flour and less grits.

Meat or game was often cooked with vegetables as a stew in large iron pots hung in fireplaces. Similar but larger iron pots with short legs were used to cook in fires outside the house. The large black cast iron pots were not only used to cook pork and fish stews but to wash clothes. For special occasions, like birthdays, whole chickens and turkeys, as well as large cuts of meat, were roasted in fireplaces or outside on open fires. Large, sharp pointed, iron rods called spits were used to hold and rotate the food. This was the beginning of southern barbecue.

The Healing Springs farmers had trouble storing food over the winter. They salted, dried, and smoked meats. Root vegetables, such as potatoes, were stored in dry, cool places, like under houses or in potato stacks made of straw and covered with dirt.

Coffee, tea, and hot chocolate were becoming popular drinks in the late 1700s and being used more and more by farmers. In the early days, most farmers ate cold meat and bread with coffee for breakfast and supper. Dinner, a large cooked meal with meat, bread, and vegetables, was served about midday or early afternoon. As farmers became wealthier and had more food to consume, all three meals were cooked.

Most of the furniture in the Boylston home was made by William and George, except for a few pieces Alice owned when she got married. The kitchen table was made of wide oak boards resting on stands like saw horses. After each meal the table was placed against the wall to provide more space. Wooden benches were used on each side of the table. Initially there was only one chair in the house, for William's use at the head of the table. (It was with this practice the term "chairman of the board" originated. Many early homes had only one chair.) As wealth increased, better furniture was added. Eventually there would be numerous chairs. However, the children would continue for generations using benches during meals.

The most popular chests of drawers were "highboys" and "lowboys." The highboys were used in bedrooms while lowboys were used in other rooms. Tall cupboards were placed in halls and in the kitchen.

Beds were made from large wooden planks and slats. Children used cots or bunk beds. Mattresses and pillows were filled with cotton or feathers. Both men and women wore nightgowns—the men called theirs nightshirts. Of course, both men and women wore nightcaps when the weather was cold. The only heat in the house was usually one fireplace.

Women on the farms worked as hard as the men. In addition to helping with the planting, harvesting, raising chickens, and milking cows, they cleaned house, cooked, wove fabrics for clothes, sewed, washed clothes, and cared for the sick. All this was done while bearing a child almost every year during their child-bearing years. It was these early farm wives and mothers who coined the phrase, "A man works from sun to sun, but a woman's work is never done." Women usually wore wool, linen, or cotton dresses; a petticoat; and a single undergarment called a shift. When outdoors in winter, women wore large capes with hoods.

Farmers wore britches and long linen or cotton shirts in the summer. In winter, they wore woolen or leather britches, knitted stockings, and heavy leather shoes. When outside in winter, they wore large loose fitting overcoats, leather leggings, woolen mittens, and a fur or leather cap. Children usually wore clothing similar to that of their parents.

Concern about disease was constant, especially for children, since there was usually no medicine to treat illness. Most large families living near Healing Springs, like the Boylstons, lost one or more children to various diseases. George and Alice's first daughter, Annie, died in 1792, during the first year of her life, from disease. There was no treatment for measles, smallpox, typhoid fever, bubonic plague, or yellow fever. The first use of the smallpox vaccine in America was by William Boylston's cousin, Dr. Zabdiel Boylston, in Boston in 1721. Settlers suffered from other serious diseases including dysentery, gout, influenza, pneumonia, rheumatism, scurvy, and tuberculosis. Generally herbs, barks, and roots were the only forms of medicine. Some quinine was available to treat malaria, called ague. The most popular medicines were made from tobacco leaves and the roots of the ginseng plant and sassafras tree. Doctors, for the most part, did not exist in the Backcountry of South Carolina.

Despite the hardships, illnesses, and wars, Backcountry settlers around Healing Springs continued to improve their lives and accumulate wealth. This was especially true for those farmers like the Boylstons who turned to growing cotton after the Revolutionary War.

William died in 1791. Within five years after their arrival in Healing Springs, the George Boylstons had outgrown their log cabin. They saved most of their profits from cotton production and had enough money to build a new, larger home. It was to be located on high ground near the cabin in a grove of large oak trees. The cabin later served as a home for George and Alice's children.

By 1795 a number of water powered sawmills had been built by the Walkers and other families along dammed streams near Healing Springs. George cut down large pine and oak trees on the property and hauled the logs by oxen to the sawmill. There, the logs were cut into boards and beams. William, who was an excellent carpenter, had taught George well. As payment for sawing the logs, the sawmill owner kept about one fourth of the lumber.

With the knowhow, necessary resources, and location, George was ready to build their home. He had the blueprint in his head. Like the Reed house, the Boylstons' would be among the first two-story clapboard homes built near Healing Springs. To ensure it would remain high and dry, the house would rest on brick pillars about five feet tall. The brick was hauled by wagon from Charles Town.

A wide porch, high off the ground, would extend across the front of the house, positioned to get only morning sun. A large, separate kitchen, behind the house, would be connected by a covered porch running the length of the house. A wide center hall would run the length of the house, from front to back. Two large rooms with fireplaces would sit on each side of the hall.

The front room on the left would be the parlor that Joanna and Alice insisted they have; the back room on the left was Joanna's bedroom. Large windows would open onto the back porch and beside the chimney. Across the hall from the bedroom would be a large dining room, with large windows like the bedroom. The front room on the right would be a bedroom for the small children. Later, it would serve as a guest bedroom.

Oak stairs would lead from the center hall upstairs to the four bedrooms. A center hall would extend through the house like downstairs. The hallways would catch any available breeze and cool the house during the summer. Ceilings would be ten feet high, which would also help cool the house. As today, settlers in South Carolina were more concerned about cooling homes than heating them. That's why most bedrooms did not have fireplaces.

The new house would feature a large brick chimney on each side and another chimney for the kitchen. There would be two large windows in every room and at each end of the upstairs hall. Wide oak steps would lead to the front porch. Even though the house would perch five feet off the ground, the porch would have no rails. Back steps would descend from the covered porch and connect the house to the kitchen.

Prior to building the new house, George dug a well near the back porch so a hand pump could be installed on the porch. There, a counter would be installed where buckets and pans could be filled with well water. Also, washbasins would be placed there for washing faces and hands in the mornings and before meals. A peg on a nearby post would hold a towel. Another peg would hold a gourd dipper for drinking.

When the first log cabin was built, William and George dug a pit and built a one-hole outhouse behind the cabin near the barn. As the family grew, it became obvious a one-holer would not be sufficient. George decided a four-holer was needed for the new house. A much larger pit was dug and a large two-door outhouse was built over the pit. A wall was built inside the outhouse, separating it in half, allowing use by both women and men simultaneously. This was quite an accomplishment and well received by all. Old cornshucks and corncobs were widely used as "toilet tissue." It would be many years before paper would find its way into outhouses—and then in the form of pages torn from old Sears Roebuck catalogs. One catalog would last an average farm family many months.

George had everything ready—the well, house design, lumber, pegs, nails, and split wood shingles. Now what was needed was time and labor. He would begin construction in May, after the April rains and before the weather got too hot. The Healing Springs community, like most rural communities at that time, helped each other out with planting, harvesting, and building barns and homes.

Once the neighbors learned of George's plans to build a new home, they offered their assistance. They were glad to do so, since they knew George was an excellent carpenter and he would help them with their buildings.

When the day arrived for the Boylstons' house-raising, about thirty-five men, twenty-five women, and fifty children showed up. They arrived soon after sunrise in a caravan of wagons, buggies, and horses. The men brought their handsaws, crosscut saws, hammers, axes, planers, and other tools. The women brought baskets of food of all descriptions and immediately set up outside cooking and eating areas under the large oak trees.

Since George had constructed the brick pillars to support the house weeks before, the foundation was ready. Most of the men assisting with the house-raising had done it before and moved quickly and efficiently. Once the floor beams and joists were in place, heart pine floors were installed. Such floors, usually two inches thick would last hundreds of years. By noon, the entire first floor had been framed. The women began serving dinner, the big midday meal: ham, chicken, vegetables, cornbread, biscuits, gravy, pies, cakes, milk, and cool Healing Springs water.

The house-raising continued until dark. By then, the entire house was framed and ready for the shingles on the roof and clapboards on the side. Everyone headed for home with buckets of leftover food. They would return about a week later for one more day, during which the house would be finished on the outside. In the meantime, George and hired labor would complete the bracing of the walls, begin installing the chimneys, and frame the windows and doors. After the clapboard siding and shingles were in place and the chimneys completed, George would finish the windows, doors, outside trim, and interior walls and ceilings. This would take the remainder of the summer, working between farm chores. The family was able to move into its new home, named Oak Grove, by September.

Since settlers first arrived in the Healing Springs area, there had been a problem obtaining enough labor. As Capt. John Smith proclaimed a hundred years earlier, "This country is long on land and short on men." Farm work was labor intensive. Thus, there was no other choice for the farmers than to work hard. One solution to their labor shortage was to have large families. Children worked as soon as they were old enough. There were no questions then about the use of child labor.

The Healing Springs middle class farmers represented the backbone of the state and nation—strong, fearless, independent people, simple in taste, democratic in social relations, defensive of their rights, sensitive to encroachments on their liberties, and earnest, narrow, and dogmatic in their religion.

The early trader-settler period of Healing Springs ended December 23, 1794, when Nathaniel Walker, Sr., died. He was buried near Walker Station in the family cemetery.

TRANSPORTATION

The Healing Springs community was still hampered by poor roads in the late 1700s. The roads, which had not advanced much beyond the widened wilderness Indian trails, were rough, muddy, and sandy and had few bridges. Notches cut on trees along the trails, to mark the way, were still visible. Many of the roads became known as "Two Notch Road" or "Five Notch Road." Ferries were still used to cross most large rivers. Some travelers declared the South Carolina roads the worst in the world. No effort was made to grade or surface the roads, or provide drainage or signs. It was not unusual for travelers to lose their way on the endless trails of dreary pines, sandy barrens, and dismal swamps. The roads were dusty in summer and muddy in winter.

Travelers through the South Carolina Backcountry usually had many miles to travel between stops. Over time, these stops became inns and villages. Farmers brought commodities for sale to the inns and stagecoach stops. Often barter was used for exchange since money was scarce. After 1690, paper money was issued by the colonies. However, the value of the "bills of credit" quickly depreciated. Commodity money, such as that from corn, sheep, cattle, furs, wheat, flour, rice, tobacco, and rum, was usually used.

By the mid 1700s stagecoaches had begun to travel through the Backcountry, with Walker's trading post being one of the stops near Healing Springs. These early stagecoaches had four simple benches, three inside for nine passengers. A front bench held the driver and a tenth passenger. Eight wooden poles, four on each side, supported a light roof. Curtains, rolled up and hung on each side and in the rear, were used during cold or rainy weather. Luggage was stored under each passenger bench, which had no back. Passengers entered and exited at the front, over the driver's bench. Because of the poor roads, stagecoaches were not generally used until after 1800.

Stagecoach inns and traveler's rest stops were generally primitive and not very comfortable. An Englishman traveling through the South Carolina Backcountry wrote, "They were mostly log huts, or a frame weatherboard; the better sort consisted of one story and two rooms; the more numerous having no internal divisions . . . one corner of the room would be occupied by a pinewood chest, the family clothes press and larder; a third would be railed off for a bar, containing a rum-keg and a tumbler. The rest of the furniture consisted of two chairs and a table, all in the last stage of palsy. . . . If hunger and fatigue compelled you to remain, a little Indian corn for your horse, a blanket on the hearth, with your saddle for a pillow, to represent a bed, were the most you would obtain. . . . As to edibles, whether you called for breakfast, dinner, or supper, the reply was the same—egg and bacon. . . . Often you cooked your own meal . . . as you ate, the large wolf-breed house dog looked at you. The young children, never less than a dozen, at the smell and sight of the victuals would let up a yell enough to frighten the wolves."

Poor transportation meant poor communications. News of the outside world was slow coming to the Walkers, Reeds, Odoms, Boylstons, and others living near Healing Springs. As travelers returned from Charleston (name changed from Charles Town in 1783) they brought the news. Stagecoaches carried copies of Charleston newspapers, which were left at stagecoach stops and traveler's rests. Those living nearby, who could read, walked or rode to the stops and read the newspaper. They didn't care if the papers were a week old, since all of it was news to them. Important information spread by word-of-mouth through the community, usually at church meetings or social gatherings. It was this way they learned in 1788 that South Carolina had become the eighth state to ratify the United States Constitution. Backcountry men were not sure they liked a strong federal government. Newspapers reported the Northwest Ordinance of 1787, which created the Northwest Territory free of slavery and eventually five new states. In 1791 they learned the pleasing news that the Bill of Rights had been approved to protect them against abuse by an overbearing federal government.

The most exciting news for William Boylston came in 1789—Gen. George Washington was elected the first president of the United States. Proud of his old friend, William promptly prepared a letter to President Washington congratulating him on his election and offering his service. Washington remained in office until 1797, when he retired.

In 1800 *The South Carolina Weekly Gazette* reported the election of Thomas Jefferson as president. Jefferson was well liked by small American farmers. A few years after his election, Jefferson negotiated the Louisiana Purchase, acquiring from France for $15 million 828,000 square miles, which doubled the size of the United States.

It is hard to believe that while Healing Springs farmers still struggled along wilderness trails in the late 1700s, ships were sailing around the world (Magellan's *Victoria* the first in 1522); steam-powered road vehicles had been invented in France by Nicolas Cugnot in 1769; another Frenchman, Pilatre de Rosier, had flown in a lighter-than-air balloon in 1783; and John Fitch had built the first steamboat in the United States in 1787. In many respects the Backcountry was still a wilderness.

In the mid 1700s, South Carolina established a number of commissions to maintain public highways. Through serving on the road commission, citizens learned how the government operated. After 1800 private investors began to build hard-surfaced roads including some covered with board planks. Tolls were charged for travel over these plank roads.

HEALING SPRINGS
BAPTIST CHURCH

During the mid 1700s settlers from Scotland, Ireland, France, Germany, and Switzerland brought their own religions to the colonies. And although there were numerous religious sects in the country at the time, the colonists were still taxed to support the Anglican Church of England.

When Anglican Nathaniel Walker founded Edisto Church in the Healing Springs area in 1772, he discovered the Anglicans were not interested in establishing churches in the Backcountry. By 1763, many Baptists had moved into South Carolina's interior and, when Edisto opened its doors, about half of all Baptists in the colony lived in the Backcountry. Over the next eight years, that figure increased to seventy percent. Edisto Church likely included many faiths, but the Baptists dominated and it was logical they would assume a leadership role. Following the Revolutionary War, the Anglican Church tax ended and the Baptist movement expanded more rapidly.

During the first ten years after the founding of Edisto Church, Nathaniel Walker served as pastor. As more settlers moved into the area, membership grew so fast a new log church became necessary. The original structure stood on Walker land not far from South Edisto River. With more church members coming from across a wide area, a centralized location was desired. After much debate,

Walker offered to give the church land near Healing Springs that he had bought from the Edisto Indians.

In 1787 Nathaniel Walker, likely the church founder's son, was pastor and applied for membership in the Charleston Baptist Association. Edisto Church was then known as Regular Baptist Church.

Most Regular Baptist members were not wealthy. They were typically small farmers, such as the Boylstons and Reeds. At that time, two-thirds of all Baptists in South Carolina lived in the Backcountry and owned no or very few slaves. However, many Lowcountry Baptist plantation owners owned slaves. Some of the wealthy Baptist preachers were slaveowners—a few owned as many as twenty-seven. People differed widely in their opinions on slavery.

Those few slaves in the Healing Springs community were encouraged to attend local churches. They usually sat upstairs in the balcony or at the rear. Many were assigned duties by their owners, like helping to build and maintain the church and yard. Slaves were listed on church membership roles as "men of colour." One such slave member continued attending Healing Springs Baptist Church after being freed at the end of the Civil War. He attended each Sunday service, sitting near the front of the church, until his death in 1920.

In 1804, the Regular Baptist Church congregation was incorporated as "The Baptist Church in Christ of the Healing Springs in the Barnwell District." From that time on, the church was officially known as Healing Springs Baptist Church.

During the early to mid 1800s, Healing Springs Baptist Church membership grew so much three separate church buildings were built. The final, and existing, church sanctuary was constructed in 1853 by slave labor on high ground about 100 yards north of the springs. According to Sally Ray, a church historian, Israel Walker (a descendent of founder Nathaniel Walker) designed and helped build the existing church. Thomas All's sawmill cut the logs into wide boards and timber. The timbers were hewn by slaves with broad axes. The wide boards were hand planed. The church was built on a brick foundation, with four brick columns supporting the front portico. All the bricks were made by hand nearby. In the finished church, slaves sat along the sides and in the back.

According to Healing Springs Baptist Church records, the first log church built near the springs was about 1780. That church burned and the third church was built at the same location. A fourth church building continued to be used by colored members to 1842. The first mention of building the current church building appeared in the May 5, 1855, minutes. This structure was completed in 1857. The Healing Springs Academy, built between the church and the springs in the 1840s, operated for many years.

The importance of Healing Springs Baptist Church to the community and county cannot be overemphasized. Farming was grueling work in the early years of the colony. It demanded the full attention of every able-bodied man, woman, and child, seven days a week. Except for chores that could not be ignored, like feeding livestock, farm families rested on Sundays. Early Sunday morning they attended church. After the church service, in summer, there was often "dinner on the grounds." Every family brought food, usually cooked on Saturday, and put it out on long tables covered with white tablecloths. One table was spread with meats, such as fried chicken, ham, and turkey. The next table held all types of vegetables, most fresh from home gardens. By July there was fresh corn, peas, okra, beans, squash, turnip greens, and potatoes—both Irish and sweet. Another table held fresh baked bread including biscuits, cornbread, and rolls. As always, near the bread were many different types of jellies, jams, and preserves including blackberry, peach, pear, plum, and watermelon rind. Close by were jugs of sugar cane syrup.

The best was saved for last. On the end table under a big oak tree was the most beautiful sight: a table covered with every kind of cake, pie, pudding, and fruit cobbler imaginable. Chocolate cake went fast. And the sweet potato and blackberry pies were rapidly consumed. Not far from the dessert table was a large wooden barrel filled with fresh, cool Healing Springs water. Everyone brought their own tin cups, which they filled many times during dinner.

Once the meal was over the women and teenage girls put the food away and cleaned the dishes at the springs. The men put the tables in the storage shed behind the church. Members continued to socialize into the afternoon. Usually, the men not attending church conference meetings gathered under one of the large oak trees and discussed the weather and farming, as well as community, state, and national affairs. In the mid 1860s, much of the discussion was about the gathering storm over slavery. In general, Healing Springs Baptists were, as they had always been, lukewarm about the subject. Few of them owned slaves but they understood that large farm and plantation owners needed extra labor. They did not feel the slavery problem was important enough to secede from the Union. However, they were independent minded and believed that South Carolina had the right to secede if it wanted to—for whatever reason. The colonies had seceded from Britain, why not South Carolina from the United States?

While these farming and political discussions took place among the men, the women talked of family and community concerns. A major topic was sickness and how to treat illnesses. They also discussed upcoming births, engagements, and marriages. Conversations remained caring, polite, and civil, as gossip was frowned upon by the Baptists.

The greatest activities after dinner were those of the young adults and children. Church was about the only opportunity young adults had to meet each other and court. As soon as the young women finished their work clearing tables, they gathered under one of the trees. Soon the young men joined them. After polite conversation, a number of them began to pair off and stroll down the path toward the springs. As they walked, their conversation turned to those things young people have talked about for thousands of years. If the day was really hot, they would take their shoes off and wade in the cool spring water. Then they would select a large rock or log nearby where they sat and continued courting until about

3:00 P.M. when the church bell rang, indicating it was time to go home.

As the young adults courted, the children ran, jumped, shouted, and played. Older children separated themselves, with boys playing rough and tumble games such as crack the whip, while the girls played hopscotch. It was a chance for children to play with kids other than their siblings. Over time, these children would grow into young adults, enter the courting phase, and eventually marry, having known each other all their lives.

Early pastors of Healing Springs Baptist Church included Nathaniel Walker, the founder, 1772-1794; James Sweat, 1795-1805; Henry Hand, 1806-1809; Thomas De Loache, 1810-1820; Darling Peeples, 1821-1846; B. W. Whilden, 1847-1848; Lucius Cuthbert, 1857-1858; and S. B Sawyer, 1858-1869.

Healing Springs Baptist Church records show that members in 1823 included Rhubin Thomas, Israel Walker, William Matheny, John Walker, Jessie Lee, John Baxley, N. Walker, and the families of Johnson, Ives, Reed, Peeples, Thomas, Odom, Bloom, Elkins, Boylston, and others. In 1836 George Boylston's youngest son, Austin, was appointed to a church committee and served as a delegate to the Association meeting.

There are only two graves at Healing Springs Baptist Church, those of Mrs. M. E. Minus and her daughter Cora. Both died in 1882. Minutes of the April 25, 1884, church conference recorded a discussion forbidding additional burials on church grounds for fear it would harm the springs. On July 26, 1884, it was decided that "no personal persons" would afterward be buried on the church grounds. On January 11, 1896, Mrs. Julia Carroll donated an acre of land adjoining the Old Walker Burial Ground to Healing Springs Baptist Church to be used for burial. The land, however, was never officially deeded to the church. Today, it is known as Seventeen Pines Cemetery.

Members of Healing Springs Baptist Church discussed many times the need for a baptismal font or pool. In August 1900, Mrs. Boylston, who owned the springs, planned to build a bathing pool and offered to let the church use it for baptism. The brick wall of the pool remains today on Windy Hill Creek east of and directly behind the church. This property was formerly owned by Nancy Boylston.

COTTON AND SLAVES

Early man was a keen observer of nature and learned that animal and plant fibers could be spun into thread and the threads twisted into rope and woven into cloth. Wool from sheep was one of the first animal fibers used. Not long after, flax plants were used to make linen. Once it was understood how to use fibers to spin thread, people were on the lookout for other fibers they could utilize. One such early fiber was cotton. The Aztec Indians cultivated cotton for textile purposes about 8,000 years ago in Mexico. Asiatic cotton grew wild in East Africa about 5,000 years ago and was used to spin thread for clothing, rope, and harnesses. Early Greeks and Romans described cotton plants as the fleece of little lambs growing on plants. Alexander the Great's army was the first to bring cotton textile goods into Europe in the 300s B.C.

The first cotton cloth was so expensive only the very rich could afford it. However, the Moslems eventually brought cotton textile manufacturing to Spain and Italy. From there, cotton processing spread throughout Europe. The English began to import cotton in the 1600s from the Mediterranean area for processing in English textile mills. In the eighteenth century, as demands for cloth increased, English textile inventors Hargreaves and Arkwright designed better yarn-manufacturing machines. The increased yarn supply expanded weaving capacity. Cartwright, another English textile inventor, then invented the power loom to speed the weaving of cloth. The Industrial Revolution in England had begun.

A tremendous supply of cotton was needed to feed the English textile mills. English merchants searched the world over for new sources of cotton. Once the American colonies were established, they became a potential source of supply, so cotton planting was encouraged. About the time the American Revolution ended, there were early attempts by southern farmers to grow cotton. They realized cotton could become a moneymaking product. The first bale of American cotton reached Britain in 1783.

Production was slow in the beginning because it was difficult to remove the seeds from the upland short-staple green-seed cotton. More and more labor was needed to remove the seeds—this labor was supplied by slaves. The number of slaves in South Carolina increased proportionally with cotton cultivation.

The year 1792 saw a great breakthrough in cotton production. Eli Whitney, while visiting Mulberry Grove Plantation on the Savannah River near Savannah, Georgia, invented the cotton gin. While a slave could remove seed from only about one pound of cotton per day, the new gin could clean about fifty pounds in the same time period. As a direct result of Whitney's cotton gin, United States cotton production rose from 140,000 pounds in 1791 to 35 million pounds in 1800.

Recognizing the potential for wealth, hundreds began moving into Barnwell District. Some set up farms along the South Edisto River. Most of these new small farmers were not slaveowners and provided their own labor.

Increased cotton production required more cleared land. The Walkers, Boylstons, and other community farmers began purchasing additional property and cutting down more trees. By this time a number of waterpowered sawmills operated on creeks leading into South Edisto River. Earthen dams and spillways were constructed with overshoots for waterwheels. These waterwheels not only powered large saws for cutting logs into lumber, but they also powered grist mills. For the next hundred years, waterwheels remained the major power source along the South Edisto River and across the state.

As farmers cleared land for cotton planting, they profited from the sale of timber, since lumber was always needed to build larger homes and barns. Healing Springs farmers enjoyed a time of increasing wealth and great opportunity.

Although few slaves were brought onto the small Healing Springs farms, hundreds were used on the large Barnwell District farms—those cultivating 2,000 to 3,000 acres. These wealthy landowners were leaders in their communities and active in local and state government.

The first slaves in South Carolina were Indians captured by the Spanish during the first year of colonization, but in the late 1700s enslaved Africans arrived from the West Indies in large numbers. Over the next twenty years, more than half of all slaves in South Carolina came from the Caribbean. Initially only a few slaves were brought to Charleston for work in Lowcountry indigo and rice fields. British merchants, during this period, began to transport slaves directly from Angola in Africa. The slave population in the state increased only about five percent per year until 1712. After that the number of slaves brought in jumped from about 100 per year to 600 per year.

African tribal chiefs captured and sold their own people to the English slave traders. The English traders branded the slaves and transported them in crowded ships to America. Because of horrendous conditions on the slave ships, many died during the voyage. Charleston was the usual destination for slave ships coming to South Carolina. Once in port, slaves were held on Sullivan's Island in quarantine before being auctioned off in the city.

In 1708, the black slave population in South Carolina exceeded the white population, with 4,080 whites and 4,100 blacks. By 1720, there were twice as many black slaves as whites. As the slave population grew, especially after the Revolutionary War, and cotton production increased, there was concern about slave rebellion. Slave codes were enacted to ensure control. By the end of the Revolution, there were still about twice as many blacks in South Carolina as whites.

It is interesting to note that in the early 1700s some blacks were armed and fought alongside the white militia against Spaniards and Indians. Most South Carolina slaveowners believed *their* slaves were loyal and trustworthy, while the *bad* slaves belonged to others. To a great degree, this is how most parents feel about their children. Later, landowners would learn the hard way they did not know how their slaves felt.

Many slaves had some control over their daily lives, especially after their chores were completed. It is to their credit that they made the best of a very bad situation and learned to cope with adversity—their very survival depended on it. Most blacks in the United States today can trace their ancestors back to these survivors.

Although still slaves, many were able to work their own gardens, fish in local ponds and streams, hunt in nearby forests, and visit neighboring plantations. They were constantly looking for some way to better their lives, soon realizing the more valuable they were to their owners, the better chance they had to improve their lot and to survive. Also, a valuable slave was likely to remain on the same plantation with his or her family. One of the best ways a slave could increase his or her value was by learning new skills, such as carpentry, iron working, cooking, weaving, animal care, and farming skills. Once they were recognized for their newly acquired skills, they requested and often received more benefits and more freedom.

In the late 1600s, abolitionists throughout the world pushed to do away with the slave trade. Quakers in England began an antislavery movement in 1671. Denmark stopped slave trade in 1792. England abolished slavery in 1833. Yielding to pressure, the United States prohibited further importation of slaves after January 1, 1808. However, the practice of slavery continued until 1865.

Not all slaves in South Carolina were passive. There were a number of slave uprisings. The first occurred in 1720 when a group of fourteen slaves planned an attack on white slaveowners. One of their own betrayed them, however, and the hunt was on to capture Primus, the leader, and his fellow slaves. After a chase through the

Backcountry, four of the group were finally captured at Savannah Town, about thirty miles from Healing Springs. The captured slaves were executed in Charleston. The next major rebellion occurred in 1739. A group of slaves met on the Stono River about twenty miles southwest of Charleston. There, they broke into a store, killed the owners, and took arms and ammunition. As these slaves proceeded toward Spanish Florida and freedom, other escaped slaves joined them, increasing their number to about 100. When they stopped to rest near present-day Jacksonboro on the Edisto River, they were discovered by no other than Lt. Gov. William Bull. He spread the alarm and a fight ensued. Fourteen slaves were killed and others captured. The remainder fled into the Edisto River swamp where most were later captured. One leader, however, hid in the swamp for three years before he was caught. This slave rebellion was the largest in British North America.

It has long been said that money is the root of all evil. Slavery in South Carolina was an example of this. Wealthy landowners saw an opportunity to greatly increase their profits by buying slaves, the only ready source of farm labor in South Carolina. Their greed for greater profit led them down the dark path of slavery. As more and more slaves were used, private citizens, government, and churches accepted the practice. Since slaveowners were leaders in local and state government and in churches, there were few willing to speak out against slavery. It was this minority of very powerful slaveowners, protecting their profits, that led the South into the Civil War.

THE IN-BETWEEN YEARS

The period between the end of the Revolution and the beginning of the Civil War was an interesting time for America.

In 1789 the French Revolution began and George Washington was inaugurated president of the United States. Most people around Healing Springs paid little attention to the news from France. They were more concerned with putting their lives back in order after the bloody American Revolution. However, they did take notice in 1803 when the latest newspaper from Charleston revealed that President Jefferson had bought all of the Louisiana territory from Napoleon Bonaparte for $15 million. This purchase from France doubled the size of the United States. Even before the purchase was complete, Jefferson sent Lewis and Clark to map the region and travel to the Pacific Ocean. The thought of all that new land excited many in the Healing Springs community, and young men set out for the South and West where they could obtain large tracts of land for little money.

The Healing Springs Baptist Church also noted the second great religious awakening of 1790. This movement was similar to the first awakening about fifty years earlier, which led to the founding of the Edisto Church by Nathaniel Walker. This time, however, the Methodists were taking a leadership role. A great camp meeting was held the summer of 1790 at Healing Springs. A number of preachers traveled from miles around to the camp meeting. People brought tents and camped for days. Services were held all through the day and into the night around a campfire. There was music and singing. Local slaves also attended the camp meetings and many were converted.

These 1790 camp meetings were the beginning of many such camp meetings in the years to come, held at Healing Springs and on the South Edisto River. Some of these meetings were held into the late 1920s. The remains of some of the campgrounds and shelters can still be seen near Boylston Landing on South Edisto River, not far west of old Holman's Bridge. The camp meetings were similar to dinners held on the grounds of Healing Springs Baptist Church, except the camp meetings lasted for days at a time. These "revivals" brought a sense of uplift and comfort to farm families, as well as the slaves, attending.

As the religious camp meetings were taking place, war broke out between Great Britain and France. In the beginning, the United States benefited from the war by exporting more agricultural products to Europe. American farmers and shippers profited. In 1805 the British navy began to stop American ships and impress thousands of sailors and passengers. John Quincy Adams, son of President John Adams, proclaimed the action an authorized system of kidnapping upon the ocean. There were many verbal exchanges between the U. S. and Britain until 1807, when a British frigate fired on a U. S. warship in American waters. This act forced Jefferson into action. He pushed through Congress the Embargo Act, which prohibited American ships from trading with foreign ports and stopped the export of American goods. Exports dropped from $108 million in 1807 to $22 million in 1808. During that same period imports also fell from $145 million to $58 million. The entire nation suffered from the Embargo Act—the New England shippers hurt the most. Farmers around Healing Springs were also hurt, but they could live off their farms and store nonperishable goods, such as cotton, until the Embargo Act was rescinded. Realizing the great harm to Americans, Jefferson called an end to the embargo. During his final week in office, in early 1809, Congress repealed the Act.

President James Madison tried to improve the situation, but in June 1812 he was finally pressured into declaring war on Britain. Thus began the War of 1812. When this news reached Healing Springs, area residents found it difficult to understand the government's action. They wondered why the nation would want to become involved in another war with Great Britain. Things were just beginning to improve after the last war. For the most part, these farmers continued their lives as usual, with little concern about the war. This was not the case, however, elsewhere in the nation—a nation unprepared for war. The American army was small and ill qualified for battle. The British blockaded the East Coast. An American invasion of British-owned Canada failed, but the navy won a victory on Lake Erie. Then Tecumseh led an Indian attack against the Americans. This attack concerned Healing Springs settlers, since there were still many Indians in Georgia, western South Carolina, and North Carolina.

Then, the bad news arriving from Charleston got

worse. The British burned the White House and captured the nation's capital city of Washington. Backcountry residents were concerned the British would head south like they did during the Revolutionary War. Perhaps remembering how things turned out in the Backcountry during the last war, the British chose only to blockade Charleston and Savannah. The British decided to end the war before Gen. Andrew Jackson's victory at New Orleans. In the end there was nothing gained, but much lost by both sides. America became determined to stay out of European wars.

Most area farmers in the early 1800s did not own enough land to provide their children with farms of their own when they married. Not only was this due to small farm acreage, but the large number of children. Couples, like George and Alice Boylston, began having children while in their early twenties and continued to do so for close to twenty years. Families often included nine or ten children. Since parents usually lived until they were in their 60s, their oldest children would have married and started their own families many years before the parents died. Shortage of family land required most older children to move to other parts of the county or state—or even to other states—and start their own homesteads. Most of George and Alice's sons left the Healing Springs area, for Georgia, Alabama, and Florida.

Usually, older sons accumulated savings to buy their own land and farm equipment by sharecropping on the parent's land or by working for neighboring farmers. Once they saved about a third of the value of the property they wanted to purchase, they mortgaged the remainder. Some rented small farms until they saved enough to buy their own.

Mothers, wives, and daughters were the glue holding families together, both economically and morally. They worked continuously, except for Sunday socials at the church. They wove fabrics and sewed clothes, cooked, made soap, churned butter, milked cows, helped in the fields, washed and ironed clothes, cleaned house, canned or otherwise preserved food, took care of the children, and helped neighbors as needed. Despite their great contributions, women had few legal rights—and, once married, usually lost control of their dowry. In most cases, the land given to young women by their families became the property of their husbands after they married. In a few cases, if there were no children when a married daughter died, the property she and her family owned before her marriage was returned to her family. This was called a "fee conditional."

Following the War of 1812, the price of most agricultural commodities rose substantially. Healing Springs farmers were tempted by the high prices to sell more of their crops for profit. This was the beginning of a market economy, which continues today. The venture into growing crops for profit also led to the need to borrow money and, in turn, an influx of bankers. The debts eventually hurt small farmers, when the prices of their crops dropped or there was a drought.

In 1818 the territory of Missouri applied for admission to the Union. This addition would upset the balance of slave versus free states. North and South were clearly defined in the east, but no such line of separation existed in the west. There was heated debate in Congress and southern newspapers carried the stories. As the debate continued, the North and South became more polarized. Finally, the Missouri Compromise was reached in 1820. Maine would enter the Union as a free state to maintain the balance, with slavery banned north of the southern boundary of Missouri, except for Missouri. This was the beginning of many such battles in Congress over slavery— battles that would not end until the Civil War.

In 1819, the western land boom collapsed sending a financial panic throughout the nation. A credit squeeze drove down the prices of corn, cotton, and tobacco. Cotton prices plunged from thirty-two cents a pound in 1818 to seventeen cents a pound in 1820. During this period many farmers lost their farms in foreclosure to banks. In an effort to help the farmers, higher tariffs were passed in 1824 and 1828.

In 1828, almost a decade after the Missouri Compromise, Healing Springs farmers faced another problem. The Charleston newspapers reported the passing of a new tariff by Congress favoring the rising industrial interests of the North and harming the agricultural exports of the South. Senator John C. Calhoun of South Carolina took up the southern cause, declaring the tariff would be nullified by South Carolina or the state would secede. In 1832 Congress passed another tariff, which South Carolina also declared null and void. President Andrew Jackson asked Congress for the power to enforce the tariffs in

South Carolina. When cooler heads prevailed, some relief for the tariffs on agricultural products was obtained and the crisis was defused. However, the talk of secession continued.

South Carolina farmers were trapped in a market economy. They would have to adjust and learn how to maximize their profits and minimize their losses. It was vital for Healing Springs farmers to get their crops to market as soon as possible after harvesting. A faster and less expensive method of transportation was needed. Barges down the Savannah and Edisto Rivers were not satisfactory. Use of the Savannah River meant that many agricultural products ended up in Savannah, Georgia, rather than in Charleston. Obviously, the Charleston merchants were concerned and searched for a way to channel more Backcountry products their way. Their solution: improving the roads and building new canals and more bridges on the waterways.

THE RAILROAD

The Industrial Revolution in England and then in the United States fueled many inventions, including machines powered by water and steam. John Fitch built the first steamboat in America in 1787, and in 1807 Robert Fulton's steamboat chugged up the Hudson River. No more than 60 steamboats used the Mississippi River in 1820. By 1846 there were 1,200. It seems a logical move from water transportation to land vehicles powered by steam, and in 1804—less than twenty years after the first steamboat—Richard Treovithick of England invented the first steam railway locomotive. By 1825, England enjoyed regularly scheduled train services and John Stevens in Hoboken, New Jersey, had tested a steam locomotive for use in America.

When news of the new railroad steam engines reached Charleston merchants, they were quick to see the opportunities this mode of transportation presented. Steam engines could be used to haul agricultural products from the interior of South Carolina. The charter for the South Carolina Canal and Railroad Company was established in 1827. To divert traffic away from Savannah the railroad was extended from Charleston to Hamburg, South Carolina, located across the Savannah River from Augusta, Georgia. This railroad was the longest in the world at that time and cost $600,000.

News of the railroad spread throughout Barnwell

County. Small Healing Springs farmers realized the advantage in getting their products to Charleston and receiving manufactured goods more rapidly. When the railroad surveyors began to travel through the area, there were many questions. Soon they were laying out the 140-mile route.

While small farmers were generally pleased about the new mode of transport, some large farmers were concerned. They had already established relatively low-cost boat transportation down the Savannah River. Some even complained the noise from the locomotives would disturb the area's peace and quiet.

In 1830, once the proposed route was laid out, construction of the railway line began. A steam locomotive purchased for $4,000 from a New York foundry would be placed in service as soon as the tracks were completed. The project was well-organized and proceeded on schedule.

John Alexander Black of Charleston headed up the railroad's Committee of Inquiry and was a driving force in the venture. He was responsible for determining the railroad's final route. His engineers and surveyors decided to run the line through the existing village of Barnwell, the oldest settlement in the district. A water and fuel stop would be located there. Col. Barney Brown, Barnwell's most prominent citizen and a large landowner, refused to sell his land for a railroad right-of-way, claiming the railroad would be too noisy and dangerous for a respectable community.

Colonel Brown's objections resulted in Alexander Black instructing his engineers to route the railroad about ten miles north of Barnwell toward Healing Springs. The small farmers there were delighted. They recognized the importance of the railroad and welcomed the opportunity to have it nearby. The railroad line ran through present-day Blackville where a water and fuel stop was established. Since trains leaving Charleston would reach Blackville about dark and not continue until daylight, as they had no lights and engineers could not see obstructions, this stop became an overnight stop.

There were few houses near the train stop. Some passengers lodged at the nearby home of Cornelius Tobin. Built in the late 1700s, this imposing house, called Fairmount, was as splendid as any structure in Charleston, and the grounds included a crude golf course.

The railroad construction camp eventually developed into the town of Blackville. Both whites and black slaves helped build the railroad bed. As construction proceeded, wooden shacks replaced workers' tents. Descendants of these early railroad workers, white and black, still live in the Blackville area.

In 1830, during construction of the Charleston-to-Hamburg railroad line, there were still Indians living in nearby swamps and woods. One surveyor writing to his nephew about the rudimentary living conditions told of the Indians. He said there were only three white men living in the area. Barnwell County's Edisto Indians were likely the first red men in America to see steam locomotives.

When the railroad line was completed in 1833, the first train to travel the entire route, the *Phoenix*, pulled out of Charleston on its way to Hamburg. Some reports claim the *Best Friend* made this trip. The *Best Friend*, in fact, made the first run before the line was completed, but the boiler exploded and the *Best Friend* was blown to pieces.

Late in the afternoon on that first full run, the *Phoenix* rolled, huffing and puffing, into Blackville. People for miles around, including the Walkers, Reeds, and Boylstons from Healing Springs, waited by the tracks as the train approached. They had plenty of time to examine the locomotive since Blackville was an overnight stop.

This area of Barnwell County grew to prominence because of its importance as the overnight stop on the longest railroad in the world. In the beginning, the village was not impressive to the rail passengers. According to Barnwell County historical records, an early passenger who had traveled ninety miles in ten and a half hours described his trip from Charleston this way: Blackville was a rough compound with two or three log houses, a tent storehouse, and an unfinished tavern located in a half-burnt forest of pitch pine. The lodging included five rooms for twenty-five passengers. Male passengers shared rooms and beds, while women passengers shared other rooms. The fee was a pleasant four dollars for dinner, bed, and breakfast.

Blackville grew rapidly as a result of the railroad, and the passenger accommodations improved. As this town progressed, the town of Barnwell realized it had made a terrible mistake in judgement in turning the locomotive away.

As the Charleston-to-Hamburg railroad succeeded, Alexander Black decided to move from Charleston to

Blackville. When his new home was completed, he relocated his family to the village, which bore his name. Black became the village's leading citizen and a large farmer. He lived there for the remainder of his life, using the railroad to ship his cotton and produce to the Charleston market. Black was buried in the Methodist churchyard. His grave now lies under the present church.

The state of South Carolina issued a charter for the village of Blackville in 1837, with corporate limits extending one mile in all directions from the railroad depository. At that time, Martin Van Buren was president of the United States and Robert Hayne governor of South Carolina. Both were Democrats.

Up to the time of the railroad, Healing Springs was the focal point of the community. This changed when the railroad fuel and water stop was established a few miles south in Blackville. Today, an interstate highway bypassing a city would have a similar effect on growth. Businesses and housing develop toward the by-pass. In the case of Blackville in the early 1800s, many young couples chose to live in Blackville rather than build homes on outlying farms. It became a boomtown.

Railroad passengers rode from Charleston to Blackville for $4.50. It cost $10 to ship a mule. A hatbox could be shipped for 10¢ and a barrel of flour for 40¢.

Not only did the train bring rapid transportation to Blackville and Healing Springs, it brought rapid communications. Now, news from Charleston arrived in hours rather than days. This improved communication made the world seem a little smaller for area residents. Descendants of those living around Blackville and Healing Springs at that time later experienced similar communication surges with the telegraph, telephone, radio, television, and Internet. Like the rest of the county, they would witness similar transportation breakthroughs with automobiles and airplanes.

Compared to today's transportation, the first trains rolling through Blackville in the 1830s were primitive. The passenger car was little more than a wooden box with hard, uncomfortable seats. Smoke from the locomotive blew into the car on the passengers. By the time they arrived in Blackville their faces and clothing were covered with soot. Despite these problems, people flocked to the trains. They would give up comfort for speed. By 1850, passengers could ride a train from Charleston all the way to Chattanooga, Tennessee.

One of the first women to ride a passenger train in the United States was Cynthia Jowers, who later married James Bell, a railroad employee. Bell invited Cynthia, then a ten-year-old girl living on the train route, to ride with the railroad construction crew on one of the first trips on the Charleston-to-Hamburg rail line.

THE GOOD OLD DAYS

The lives of those living around Healing Springs improved significantly with the arrival of the railroad in Blackville. Not only could they sell more of their products, they had more money to buy manufactured goods. For the first time many new items were being used in homes and on farms that made life a little easier.

New families poured into the Healing Springs area and other parts of Barnwell County—among them, Lewis Malone Ayer, Sr., to the Buford's Bridge area; Capt. William Barker, a veteran of the War of 1812; Simon Brown to Blackville; the Carroll family; the Farrell family; and John Grubbs. Much larger homes were being built both in town and in the country. The local population increased substantially and church membership grew in leaps and bounds.

It seemed as if the Industrial Revolution had finally arrived in Barnwell County. Steam power moved the trains. Water power, provided by dams and ponds on most of the larger area streams, drove machinery for sawmills, gristmills, and flour mills. Water and steam also powered the new cotton gins.

Some of the news reaching farmers around Healing Springs made them uneasy. The daily Charleston newspapers told of Britain freeing all slaves between 1834 and 1840 and the worldwide abolitionist movement that was underway. Although small farmers were not directly involved with slavery, they realized slavery's importance to large farmers and plantation owners. An attack on slavery would surely lead to conflict. Someone arriving in Blackville in 1833 brought a copy of a new newspaper being published in the North, *The Liberator*. This abolitionist paper published by William Lloyd Garrison would continue advocating freedom of all slaves right up to the Civil War. A $5,000 reward was offered in Georgia for Garrison's arrest and conviction as a public enemy. What worried the non-slave owners the most was that people like Garrison might incite the slaves in South Carolina, who outnumbered the whites, to revolt. As evidenced by past revolts, the slaves killed whites at random, not just white slaveowners. All whites were concerned about their personal safety.

After the depression of 1837, thousands of immigrant workers began to flood into the United States seeking employment. Many headed to the New England cotton mills. Over one million Irishmen entered the United States between 1840 and 1850. Most of them worked in northern factories. Men, women, and children worked from thirteen to fifteen hours per day under very poor conditions. Thousands of injuries and illnesses occurred each year in the factories. Northern factory workers worked under conditions little better than those of southern slaves.

As cotton production and wealth increased, more and more young men left Healing Springs and Blackville with their accumulated money and traveled to other southern states where they could buy inexpensive land. Some reached Texas in the Mexico territory and bought ranches or cotton farms. In 1836 Americans outnumbered the Mexicans—in what is now Texas—and they revolted against the Mexicans. Although the Americans won control of Texas, Mexico would not recognize the territory as an independent republic. Mexico also warned the United States it would declare war if Texas was admitted to the Union.

The Charleston newspapers ran articles reporting President James K. Polk's desire to annex Texas. In 1845, Texas was made a state and Mexico broke off relations with the United States. In general, most people were pleased that Texas was now a state, as they knew people in Texas or had relatives there. However, it was not to be that easy. Disputes with Mexico increased over boundaries, Mexican debts, and the United States's "manifest destiny." President Polk sent Gen. Zachary Taylor into the disputed territory and a fight resulted. This initiated the Mexican War, which the United States won. As victor, the United States gained 525,000 square miles of territory including California, Nevada, Utah, Arizona, and parts of New Mexico and Colorado. Where few local citizens fought in the War of 1812, many more of the area's young men joined the Mexican War. Some of these would later return to Texas and establish new homes.

The Charleston-to-Hamburg railroad was, in 1836, the first railroad used to transport soldiers for military purposes. Marines from Charleston traveled through Blackville, where they spent the night, on their way to Hamburg to relieve Gen. Winfield Scott in the Second Seminole War.

Again in 1846, soldiers boarded the train in

Blackville during the Mexican War. However, this time it was volunteers from the Barnwell District. Capt. N. I. Walker, a descendant of Nathaniel Walker of Healing Springs, commanded them. Once in Mexico, these Blackville and Healing Springs natives fought with Robert E. Lee, Thomas J. "Stonewall" Jackson, and Ulysses S. Grant. Of the 1,000 South Carolinians who went to Mexico, forty-two percent did not return home. This conflict proved to be a training ground for the Civil War. Many of the Federal and Confederate generals received baptism under fire during the Mexican War.

The acquired Mexican territory brought problems as well as opportunities. The addition of the new territory renewed the question of the morality of slavery. This adversity between slave states and free states eventually led to the Civil War and disaster for the South.

An invention in 1846 that greatly affected the women of Healing Springs was Elias Howe's mechanical sewing machine, one of the first machines mass produced for home use. It made women's work easier—just like stoves, washing machines, and indoor plumbing would in later years.

More tin cans and containers were being used. Iron cooking stoves were replacing fireplaces. Work in the farm fields was more productive where the first McCormick reaper and other farm machinery were used. One of the most significant was the John Deere steel plow, which greatly speeded the preparation of fields for planting. Another mechanical device that brought great joy to all, and had a big impact on church socials, was the hand-cranked ice-cream freezer.

One summer day in 1848, headlines of Charleston newspapers announced that gold had been discovered in California. According to the papers, one had only to walk to the shallow creeks and pick up pockets full of gold nuggets. A number of young men, eager to get rich quick, said goodbye to their families and caught the next train to Charleston where they boarded ships for the West coast. Some of these young men were never heard from again.

Although most music heard around Healing Springs was good old Baptist hymns, more and more people were singing the songs of composer Stephen Foster. "Oh Susanna" and "De Camptown Races" were particular favorites. Over the next ten years, Stephen Foster would dominate the country's song writing.

As church membership grew, the need increased for more churches close to home. On November 8, 1846, twenty-seven members of the Healing Springs Baptist Church left to form a new Baptist church in Blackville. The group met in the home of Samuel Reed, northeast of town, until the church could be built. The Reed house still stands at its original location. The members of the new First Baptist Church were Austin Boylston, Lewis Nevils, Jesse Lancaster, Benjamin Watson, Pinckney Bloom, George F. Hartzog, William Lott, Mary Lancaster, Jane Odom, E. Chitty, Mary Reed, Jessie Nevils, Newport Head, Mary Nevils, Martha Nevils, Cynthia Nevils, John Babers, E. Bloom, Mary Williams, Elizabeth Reed, and Samuel Reed. Austin Boylston was elected clerk of the new church. Lewis Nevils and Jesse Lancaster served as deacons. Darling Peeples, who had previously pastored the Healing Springs Baptist Church, became its first pastor. The first church structure was a simple, one-room, wooden building with a porch and four columns. It stood on Clark Street, on land donated by Lewis and Martha Nevils. Austin Boylston was one of three trustees.

Pastor Darling Peeples died in 1850. The seventy-six-year old had lived an interesting life. He served in the South Carolina House and Senate, representing the Barnwell District before he was thirty, and he was the first clerk of court for the district. Peeples was one of the first to buy stock in the South Carolina Canal and Railroad Company and was granted free passage on the railroad for life. His stock was left to Furman College, the Baptist Publication Society, and the Baptist Church mission boards.

In 1849 the First Baptist Church of Blackville reported seventy-five members: fifty-eight white and seventeen black. Healing Springs Baptist Church continued to have black members until 1920. The black members of First Baptist left about the time the black Macedonia Church was organized, in 1866.

In 1852, northern newspapers began running a serial of the book Uncle Tom's Cabin by Harriett Beecher Stowe, which condemned slavery. Copies of these papers arrived in Charleston and found their way to Blackville. The publication was of little concern to the Healing Springs farmers directly, but they realized it was another step toward trouble. Not long after Uncle Tom's Cabin was published and distributed throughout the North, news arrived of the Kansas-Nebraska Act of 1854. The admission of more slave states angered the North.

By 1850, Blackville's population reached 3,000. Over the next ten years, the town became a large transportation and marketing center. The Baptists were concerned, as this growth brought with it some problems—specifically, five bars in a two-block area and gunfights. The railroad was now known as the Carolina Railroad.

CIVIL WAR

As often happens in human history, just when things are going well and the future looks bright, something occurs to change everything for the worse.

Farmers around Healing Springs were living the good life. They had nice homes, many of which now had board siding and two stories with large front porches. Food supply was in abundance.

Concern about the morality of slavery and the North's increasing opposition to it remained an undercurrent in the community of Healing Springs. Although most farmers in Barnwell County owned no slaves, they understood that large farmers and plantation owners needed the labor. Independent and self-reliant, Backcountry residents resented being told by powers far away and unfamiliar with them, what they could and could not do. Because of this, they were not so much pro-slavery as they were anti-government (Federal government), as their ancestors had been.

More and more the Barnwell County farmers were becoming economically tied to Europe. Southern agricultural products were sold overseas, while northern manufactured goods were selling to the great urban centers of the North and the West. As the population in the North increased, a large consumer market for northern factories established itself. The South purchased few manufactured goods from the North and developed no economic ties to that part of the country. As a result, the South became more isolated.

Habitation to the West expanded rapidly in the mid 1850s. From 1850 to 1860 Chicago grew from 30,000 inhabitants to 110,000. There was a great rush farther west in 1859 when gold was discovered near Pike's Peak, Colorado. While South Carolina was early in the initial building of railroads, other parts of the country were now constructing railroads with much more speed. By 1860, about one third of all the nation's railroads were in the Northwest.

The Kansas-Nebraska Act and the resulting debate on slavery led to the formation of the Republican Party, which was antislavery. Newspapers arriving from Charleston were full of articles on the fighting in Kansas over slavery. Northern abolitionists and the Emigrant Aid Society sent antislavery advocates into Kansas with Bibles and guns to make sure Kansas voted to be a free state. To counter this influx, Missouri southerners rode into Kansas on election day to vote for a slave state. There were a number of bloody clashes. Headlines in the newspapers proclaimed, "Bloody Kansas."

In 1859, abolitionist fanatic John Brown, who was involved in the Kansas fighting, led a group of eighteen men to Harper's Ferry, Virginia, to start a war against slavery. Most of his followers were killed and Brown was hung. This incident lent more fuel to the fire that was beginning to burn out of control. In the North, John Brown was enshrined as a saint.

The South now realized there would be no peaceful solution to the slavery issue.

Abraham Lincoln, a westerner, placed the slavery issue squarely before the nation when he stated in his 1858 debate with Stephen A. Douglas, "A house divided against itself cannot stand. I believe this government cannot endure permanently half slave and half free. I do not expect the Union to be dissolved—I do not expect the house to fall—but I do expect it will cease to be divided. It will become one thing, or all the other."

The Republicans won the election in 1860, because the South pulled out of the Democratic Party and ran a third-party candidate. Once the Democrats lost the support of the South and West, they could not win. The announcement of Lincoln's victory was the worst news the South could hear. Southern leaders felt the South had no other choice but to secede. There were now eighteen free states and fifteen slave states, and the South held a minority in both houses of Congress. People living around Healing Springs and Blackville felt the nation was anti-South. Most believed they had not changed, as they held the same beliefs of their fathers, but the rest of the nation had changed, and the South would have to adapt or die. Typically, southerners are slow to change and these farmers were determined to fight as long as it took to win their freedom from Federal government control.

To most, it was not a case of *what* was going to happen, but *when*. The month after Lincoln's election, South Carolina called a secession convention in Columbia. An outbreak of smallpox moved the convention to Charleston. Each day, Austin Boylston and others in the Healing Springs community met the afternoon train from Charleston and obtained a copy of the latest newspaper. Some of the wealthy large farmers of Barnwell District decided to travel to Charleston and see firsthand what was happening. These men were present on December 20, 1860, when the Secession Convention passed the ordinance of secession. There was great celebration up and down Meeting Street and in front of the Mills House. Lewis M. Ayer, Jr., from Barnwell District signed the Ordinance of Secession and served in the Confederate Congress during the Civil War.

News of secession did not reach Blackville until December 21 when the afternoon train brought the Charleston newspapers. There was no celebration in Blackville and Healing Springs, especially among small farmers. They remembered their grandfathers' descriptions of the Revolutionary War in the Backcountry—how neighbors and friends fought savagely against each other for eight years. Now they could envision this happening again. While the older people were very concerned, many of the young men were excited at the thought of going off to war. They did not yet understand the consequences of war.

By 1860, most of George and Alice Cloud Boylston's children had children of their own old enough to serve in the army. Austin and Polly's five sons were about the right age. James Wyatt, their first child and oldest son, was forty-three years old and married to Martha Corbitt of Salley, South Carolina. Wyatt and Martha had five children: Rachel, age nine; Mary, age six; Brooks, age four; Charlie, age three; and John, age one.

Samuel (Sam) Reed, Austin and Polly's second oldest

143

son was thirty-one years old and married to Elizabeth (Lizzie) Riley. They had four children: Emma, Brantley Furman, Laura, and Samuel Reed, Jr. Sam volunteered for service in 1862.

Presley Jefferson, Austin and Polly's third son, was twenty years old, unmarried, and a prime candidate for service in the army. George William was seventeen years old and likely to serve. Lucian (Lute) Austin, the youngest son and last child, was only fourteen years old and considered too young to fight. However, young teenage boys often left to join up.

The concern of the Boylstons was the same as the concern of all mothers and fathers with sons of fighting age. No parents wanted their sons to go off to war. However, they knew if it came to war their sons would likely fight as their grandfathers had done to protect their freedom. There was no thought among the small farmers about protecting slavery. No father and mother living in the Healing Springs and Blackville area would have sent their sons to war to protect the right to own slaves. However, they would fight for their belief in deciding for themselves what was best for them and to protect their families, homes, and state.

All the typical citizen could do in late 1860 and early 1861 was watch, wait, and pray. Special gatherings at the Healing Springs Baptist Church and the First Baptist Church of Blackville brought folks together to pray that the leaders of the South and North could reach an agreement where war could be avoided.

As they prayed, the news got worse. False news reports claimed black Republicans took over Washington and were taking action, like John Brown did, to free the slaves. Regardless of whether one owned slaves, everyone was afraid of a slave uprising against whites. Many slaveowners fostered this fear among southerners to gain support for secession.

As the news of the South Carolina secession spread throughout the South, other southern states began to secede. Each day, people rushed to the Blackville train station to get copies of the latest Charleston newspaper and learn of new developments.

Events proceeded rapidly. On December 26, 1860, Maj. Robert Anderson moved his Federal garrison at Fort Moultrie to Fort Sumter in Charleston Harbor. Four days later, South Carolina troops seized the Federal arsenal at Charleston. There was talk of a compromise in Washington, but it was soon realized that neither side was willing to settle. Most people still prayed for peace and there was talk of a new southern confederacy as more states debated secession.

As 1861 began, talk became action. News arrived in Blackville on January 10 that South Carolina troops fired on a Federal ship, *Star of the West*, which was trying to reinforce Major Anderson at Fort Sumter. Many thought the war had begun. When the ship withdrew, there was a general sigh of relief.

By February 1861, six southern states had withdrawn from the Union and called a meeting in Montgomery, Alabama. On February 8, a Confederate Constitution was adopted and the next day Jefferson Davis was elected Provisional President of the Confederacy. He was inaugurated on February 18.

On March 2, Blackville and Healing Springs farmers received news that the Confederate States had taken control of the military in Charleston and Gen. P. G. T. Beauregard was placed in command. This was surely a sign that war was about to begin.

A subsequent period of calm had everyone wondering what would happen next. The calm was broken on April 12, 1861, when Confederates fired on Fort Sumter before relief ships could restock the fort. News of the attack reached Barnwell County Saturday, April 13. Fort Sumter surrendered that same day. Two days later, President Lincoln issued a proclamation declaring an insurrection and calling for 75,000 volunteers. Newspapers rapidly spread the news throughout the nation. Upon learning of Lincoln's plan to invade the South, most of the southern border states sided with the Confederacy.

When President Lincoln declared a blockade of southern ports, the farmers around Blackville and Healing Springs knew they were in trouble. It was only a matter of time before cotton would stop being exported to Britain. That would end their profits—but not their lives. They could, as they had done in the past, live off their farms and wait until the war ended. All hoped for a brief war with only a few battles.

President Lincoln issued another call for 42,034 volunteers to serve for a possible three years. Southern state governors also requested volunteers to defend their respective states. The Confederate Congress signed a bill on May

3, 1861, declaring a state of war between the Confederacy and the Union. On May 7, the Confederate Congress authorized President Davis to accept volunteers for the duration of the war. On May 20, the Congress voted to move the Confederate capital from Montgomery, Alabama, to Richmond, Virginia.

Each day, more and more young men left their Healing Springs and Blackville homes and headed for army camps to volunteer. Prominent citizens formed volunteer companies—some infantry units, others cavalry and artillery. Camp Butler was established near Montmorenci, about fifteen miles west of Blackville on the Charleston-to-Hamburg railroad line. Most local volunteers were sent to Camp Butler for initial training before being assigned to active units.

Owen Barker of the Big Fork section of Barnwell District had twenty-two children, eleven by his first wife, Mary Getsinger, and eleven by his second wife, Elizabeth Lyons. Seven of his sons volunteered for service in the Confederate army. Other locals—William B. Carroll, William Alfred Gyles, and John Lafayette Hair, among them—joined artillery companies fighting on James Island near Charleston.

Three of Abraham Odom's seven sons served in Company H of the 17th South Carolina infantry. His son Wiatt was killed in 1862 at Second Manassas. That same year, son Richard died of wounds or illness. His only surviving son, William, returned home after the war and lived to 1905.

Robert Moore Willis, educated at The Citadel, raised

a company of volunteers from his hometown of Williston, named for his family. Willis, whose aunt married George Boylston, Jr., later became a captain in Lamar's Artillery Battalion and served with George and Presley Boylston.

Samuel Reed formed a company of artillery for training at Camp Butler. His Boylston cousins, Presley Jefferson and George William, were some of the first to join the unit. George became a sergeant. Others in the company included J. Wyatt Lancaster, James M. Baggett, Andrew Houser, Joseph J. Brown, James N. Walker, R. Frank Nevils, Nathaniel D. Walker, Charles H. Still, Henry Barr, Pinkney Butler, N. C. Cave, William B. Carroll, Monroe Cox, James E. Delk, Henry H. Dyches, Henry Felder, W. Patrick Hair, Henry D. Holman, James R. Hutto, Samuel P. Lott, Richard Martin, Darling P. Morris, Robert Nix, Aaron Odom, George Owens, Daniel Riley, Thomas Still, and Marmaduke Whaley. These young men represented some of the best of Barnwell County.

All of Austin Boylston's family was at the Blackville railroad station in May 1861 to bid Presley and George farewell. Many other families were there also, sending their sons off to war. Mothers and sisters cried as the men held back tears. The train headed west as arms waved from every window. Family members stood by the tracks until the train was out of sight. Slowly they boarded their wagons, buggies, and horses for the sad ride home, realizing that home would never be the same again.

Presley, who was twenty, and George, who was now eighteen, trained hard from sunrise to sunset each day.

After about three months, believing they were ready to fight, they anxiously awaited assignment to a permanent location. Their chance came in September, when they were sent to join Maj. Tom Lamar's heavy artillery battalion on James Island near Charleston. On their train ride from Montmorenci to Charleston they passed through Blackville. The train stopped briefly for water and fuel, but since the move was not announced ahead of time, there were no family members to greet them. They did have time to write a short note and give it to the stationmaster for delivery to their parents.

Since Presley and George's departure in May, the war had exploded into a widespread affair. Because of early Confederate victories at Big Bethel and Manassas, Virginia, the South became overconfident and believed the North would give up the fight. As the months progressed, it became clear the Yankees would not quit, despite their defeats. By late August, the Federals were on full attack and captured Confederate forts on North Carolina's Outer Banks. Not long after George and Presley arrived on James Island, the Federal navy, just outside Charleston Harbor, captured a Confederate blockade runner, *Alert*. In early October, there were rumors of a Federal attack on Port Royal, South Carolina.

During their first few months on James Island, Presley and George both were busy building gun emplacements and forts, including a large fort at Secessionville. Telegraph lines were run between defensive positions to enhance communication. By that time, the telegraph was in widespread use, the transcontinental telegraph having been completed in October 1861.

What the Confederates had feared most happened on November 7, 1861: the Federal navy attacked the Port Royal forts. Soon all of Port Royal Sound and the town of Beaufort were in Federal hands. There was great concern about the safety of Savannah, Georgia, and the Charleston-Savannah railroad line. It was obvious to the South that more fortifications and troops would be needed.

George and Presley, like other soldiers from Blackville and Healing Springs, wrote home often. Sisters Mary and Ellen sent news of home to their brothers. Austin and Polly wrote, but not as often as their daughters. Letters from both sides were filled with the spread of illnesses, throughout communities and camps. It was believed the increased travel during the war and contact with people from other areas caused the spread of many diseases.

In November, the *Charleston Mercury* reported that flames could be seen all along the South Carolina coast, as plantation owners burned their cotton to keep it out of Yankee hands. The *Charleston Courier* proclaimed the burned cotton would deprive the Federals of extensive spoils.

George and Presley wrote home in December about the disastrous fire that swept through the Charleston business district on December 11, 1861. Most of the damage was east of King Street near the Cooper River. That year, for the first time, the brothers did not attend Christmas service at Healing Springs Baptist Church. Homesick, they tried to get furloughs for a brief visit.

As January 1862 rolled around, it was clear to all that the war would be long and bloody. The South's only hope was for the North to tire of fighting and quit, or for Great Britain to step in and side with the South to maintain its cotton supply. More and more young men from Blackville and Healing Springs joined the Confederate army. Each Sunday at Healing Springs Baptist Church and Blackville's First Baptist Church, there were more and more vacant seats. There were reportedly a few seats vacated by young men who had not volunteered and were too ashamed to come to church.

Because of absent members and the shortage of food, Sunday afternoon dinners at Healing Springs Baptist Church had stopped. No one seemed interested in having fun while so many suffered such misery. Long prayers offered up each Sunday asked Almighty God for the protection of those fighting and the many sick. More young men from the community died from disease than in battle. Funerals seemed to take place weekly.

As Sam Reed Boylston saw most of his friends volunteer for the army, including some married men with children, he told his wife Lizzie he had to join up. He chose the cavalry since it was the elite of all the services. Sam was a good horseman and hunter. He was a natural cavalryman. Once he decided to volunteer, his younger brother Lute, who was only sixteen, decided to go with Sam to join the cavalry. When Lute reported to the recruitment station, he was told he was too young and could not serve without his father's written permission. Lute went to his father, Austin, and after a long debate with both parents, obtained written permission. With the letter in hand, Lute returned to the recruitment station and was accepted into the cavalry, to serve alongside his older brother. Watching their youngest son depart for war was one of the saddest things Austin and Polly had ever experienced.

Sam said goodbye to his wife Lizzie and their four children and rode off toward Charleston with Lute. They carried enough food with them for one night on the road. About forty miles west of Charleston they slept in a farmer's barn before proceeding the next morning to Adam's Run.

Brothers Presley and George Boylston fought with Lamar's Second South Carolina Regiment. Lamar's regiment was responsible for defending James Island near the village of Secessionville. They constructed a battery across the narrowest point of a peninsula. It was hard work in the hot humid weather and many of the new soldiers became ill. Capt. Samuel Reed would later succeed Col. Tom Lamar as commander of Company B, Second South Carolina Regiment, Heavy Artillery.

At first, news from the front arriving in Blackville and Healing Springs was generally good. Every effort was made by the Confederates to show they were defeating the Yankees. Even the battle of Shiloh, or Pittsburg Landing as it was called by the Yankees, was projected as a victory for the Confederates. There was no mention of the 10,694 killed, wounded, or missing troops. However, the news of those killed in battle later arrived home and the true story was revealed. From April 1862 through April 1865, bad news concerning the death of young men flowed constantly to their homes in Barnwell District.

While Gen. Robert E. Lee was driving General McClellan's Federal army from Richmond, the Federals at Charleston were attacking James Island. They headed directly toward the Boylston brothers' regiment during the early morning hours of June 16, 1862. George had been assigned to the ordinance department and Presley served as artilleryman, responsible for firing his cannon using a friction punch.

About 4 A.M. on the morning of the battle of Secessionville, George woke Presley and announced that a Federal attack was likely. Presley quickly dressed and reported to his cannon emplacement. There, he, George, and their cousin, Capt. Samuel Reed, waited for Federals to emerge from the early morning fog. They didn't have to wait long before they heard shots fired and men yelling. The Confederate pickets were being driven back toward the fort, the Federals hot on their heels. The Federals charged the gun emplacements. Presley was ready for them. Sam yelled to Presley to fire his charge of grapeshot point-blank at the charging bluecoats. Presley Boylston's cannon was the first fired in the Battle of Secessionville. That initial blast wiped out most of the first wave of Federals. By then there were hundreds of Confederates firing cannons and muskets at the approaching bluecoats. More Federals charged the cannon muzzles only to be forced back. These repeated attacks went on for hours before the Federals finally pulled back. Throughout the battle Presley stood by his cannon. At one point he, another soldier, and Captain Reed were all that remained of Company B. It was then that Reed was mortally wounded by a bullet passing through George's cap. Reinforcements arrived to push the bluecoats back. The Federals suffered heavy losses: 107 men killed, 487 wounded, and 89 missing. Of the Rebels 52 were killed, 144 wounded, and 8 missing. Since George and Presley had been separated, each thought the other had been killed. Later, upon meeting, the brothers embraced each other heartily and kissed.

News of the Confederate victory quickly spread to Blackville and Healing Springs. Joy was soon tempered by sorrow for the many Barnwell and Edgefield District men killed.

There was great sadness in the Reed and Boylston homes. Samuel Reed was the son of Austin's sister Elizabeth (Lizzie). Austin and Polly had named one of their sons Samuel Reed after Polly's brother. Special memorial services were held at the First Baptist Church of Blackville for Samuel Reed and other church members killed at Secessionville.

Ellen was quite a letter writer, corresponding with her four brothers in the Confederate service and with friends. Her letter dated January 20, 1862, to Presley and George described how George and Sam had been able to come home to Oak Grove for brief visits. She wrote, "Sammie arrived home last night on his way to Coosawhatchie. He will remain home until Wednesday night or early Thursday morning. He had a great deal to tell about camp life. I wish you all three could get together to talk it all over. Sammie had to stand guard for the first time last Tuesday night—that dreadful rainy night. He was relieved about three o'clock and went in the guard tent where there were as many as fifteen men asleep. He hardly had room to sit down all wet and cold. It seems that they have a harder time than you. I wish he had gone with you, but he says he likes it very well, as well as he expected. Well, Presley and George, I suppose you must have experienced a feeling that you never did before. That was when the long roll was beat and your company falling in ranks ready in a moments warning to attack in order to meet the enemy. Cousin Sammy (Reed) wrote us you all done exceedingly well, being the first time that the long roll had been beat. I am glad to hear how brave you all are. But yet it makes me almost tremble to think you were so near the battlefield. I am sorry to hear of so many of our men being killed and wounded. I believe none are our acquaintances, but yet I feel for them. God forbid that any of you may ever share the fate of poor Eubanks. So, boys, what ever you do, never rush into danger unnecessarily. I suppose if they had obeyed Colonel Jones, not one would have been killed. Always be careful to obey your officers especially on the battleground. Presley and George turn and sun your bedding often and hoist the sash in your room every day so that it may air well. Where there are so many in one room it may cause sickness if you are not careful. I hope you will miss the mumps—George especially on account of his neck. Presley, I suppose you have had the roseola? Well Pa got it down there or somewhere. We did not know what was the matter with him—he has been sick ever since George left, but is better now so that he can get about. . . .

Ma says she has two pair of woolen socks for you. She will send them the first good opportunity. . . ."

Brothers Sam and Lute Boylston, upon their arrival at Adam's Run in early 1862, were assigned to the 14th South Carolina Cavalry battalion based at McPhersonville. Their commander was Maj. John H. Morgan from Morgantown, near present-day Springfield. The battalion was to protect the Charleston-Savannah railroad line.

Ellen Boylston received a letter from a friend in Cartersville, Georgia, dated June 29, 1862, describing how she was making clothes for soldiers and visiting the Confederate camp at Big Shanty. She wrote, "I have just received a letter from Aunt C. She informs me of a recent visit to Orangeburg which she enjoyed greatly. Did you go? I wish that I could have been with her for she must have had a pleasant time. She laughs at the idea of my asking you if she had gone to the war. I expect if she could go she would make such havoc among those detestable Yankees. I do not swear Ellen dear, what lady would, but I cannot keep from saying confound them for they have been the instigators of all our national troubles. My expectations now are quite sanguine, for it is indeed encouraging to see that thus far in every engagement we have been victorious. It is certainly an evidence that God's omnipotent hand is extended over us."

Sam and Lute's first skirmish occurred on October 22, 1862, at Pocotaligo. Federal general Brannon led a force of 4,448 to destroy the tracks and bridges on the Savannah-Charleston railroad line. They were proceeding toward the town of Pocotaligo to destroy the railroad and capture Confederate military stores at the town of Coosawhatchie. Colonel Walker commanded the Confederate infantry and cavalry, meeting this Federal threat. One of the cavalry units was Major Morgan's battalion. They held the Federals in check, despite Morgan's being severely wounded. As Confederate reinforcements arrived, the battle grew larger. Slowly, the Confederates withdrew to the village of Old Pocotaligo. After a fierce fight, the Federals withdrew. The Confederates lost 163 men—21 killed, 124 wounded, and 18 missing—while the Federals lost 340—43 killed, 294 wounded, and 3 missing.

Mary Boylston wrote a letter on Monday, June 16, 1862, (likely to her brother Wyatt) describing what her brothers, Sam, Lute, Presley, and George told her about their skirmishes: "Perhaps you are aware of our dear brothers' situation. They have been in one hard battle on last Tuesday, a week. Pa got a letter from Pres last Saturday. It was written on Wednesday. He said they were daily expecting a hard battle. He said the hardest kind of fighting would be done on that island. When I think what a narrow escape they had, how thankful we ought to be to our God for his kind protection. Pres said the shells and balls fell in two or three feet of them. It is said that one of cousin Sammy's guns took the mast off one of the Yankee boats. It was so disabled another one of their steamers had to tow it away. This is one of the sad times with us constantly expecting to hear of our brothers being wounded or killed. What a sad, sad thought it is. Oh, how can we bear it? I guess you have heard of Sammy's narrow escape. They were in twenty yards of the Yankees when they were ordered to retreat. Sammy said it seemed that the balls did not miss his head over three inches. I believe they got only one man killed and some wounded. What a lonely time we have. Ellen and myself have to stay every night with Lizzie [Sam's wife]. . . . Oh, this horrid war; just think what it has done. Tell Ann, Joe Eaves died in a hospital in Richmond, Virginia. His corpse is to come on the cars tonight. His funeral will be preached at the Healing Springs Church tomorrow. What a sad night this is for their family. Some two or three others have died in the hospitals. Just think, this day six weeks ago we were all together but Sammy. I feel it is the last time. . . . I am afraid before you hear from us again; there will be sad changes in our family. Love to Ann. Write soon. From your sister, Mary."

Mary Boylston wrote (likely to her brother Wyatt) in June 2, 1862, "Oh, I do feel so sorry for the poor soldiers these warm days and particularly where the water is so bad as it is at the race grounds in Charleston. They have a great deal of sickness there. We got a letter from the boys yesterday. They are well. Presley had been in a scouting party. He was out two days and nearly three nights. He said he had a hard time of it. It was during the cool nights. Poor boys, we do not know what they have to endure. It is well we do not know it. Sammy has been in a fight at Pocotaligo last Thursday. They had a considerable brush. The Yankees came out to take possession of the Savannah Railroad. Sammy said they had to double quickly a quarter mile. When they got to the place, they had to lie down in a ditch. They lay there till the Yankees came in forty yards of them. One Yankee came out on the bridge. Some men shot at him and he fell dead. We got only two men killed and one horse. They only saw one of the enemy fall. They do not know how many more were killed. Sammy is to come home this week. I would like so much to hear him talk about it."

Many of the soldiers were ill and some were dying in army hospitals. A letter written on August 22, 1862, by Anne Boylston to her husband John Staley told of Pres and George being ill. She wrote, "We received a letter from Pa that was written Tuesday [apparently from Charleston]. He said Pres was rather worse off than the day before the Dr. applied a large blister that drew very well. Pa said if Wyatt would come down and bring Mary with him to stay a while. By Pa consenting for Mary to go, Ma thought he must be worse that night. Her and Mary went. The morning after they left, we received another letter saying Pres was about the same. George is sick yet. I am afraid he is bad. Pa wrote for us to send him a mattress. We haven't received one [a letter] since we feel uneasy tonight about them. We heard from Sammy today. He hasn't given up yet."

During the Civil War it was not unusual for family members like Austin, Wyatt, Polly and Mary to travel to nearby army camps to help sick sons and brothers. Such was the case when they rode the train to Charleston and nursed Pres and George on James Island. During those visits, the family members became exposed to many diseases and some became ill themselves.

Although the main interest of the Healing Springs

and Blackville citizens was their young men and the battles they fought, there was concern about the war in general. The newspapers arriving daily on the train from Charleston gave some insight to other events. They learned of the bloody battle on September 17, 1862, at Antietam Creek in Maryland. A few days later, they learned of President Lincoln's Emancipation Proclamation freeing the slaves in the South. Most southerners believed this was a call for a slave uprising. General Lee had been driven from Maryland and the war in the West was not going well. More and more, the South was being forced on the defensive. One thing was clear to all southern families: there would be many more names on casualty lists, more sorrow, more suffering, and more loss. Their whole world seemed to be falling down around them—and it was!

General Beauregard, Confederate hero of the attack on Fort Sumter, was assigned to the defense of Charleston in September 1862. He immediately began building up area defenses. He also looked for an opportunity to strike back at the Federals. Opportunity knocked on January 29, 1863, when concealed batteries along the banks of the Stono River fired on and captured the Federal gunboat *Isaac Smith*. The Healing Springs community was well represented in this attack—Presley Boylston fired the first shot. George worked in ordnance at Fort Johnson on James Island. In April 1863 the Federal navy attacked the Charleston area forts. George took part in defending most of these attacks.

Things were not going well back home in Healing Springs and Blackville. George's sister Ellen wrote him on

Tuesday January 30, 1863, "I suppose the fellow soldier that died was Black, he was buried on Monday at the Methodist Church in Blackville. There were only three or four to assist his father in burying him. Poor fellow had no mother to weep over him, nor close friends to help lay him down in the silent grave after he was brought home. I reckoned you have heard Mr. Mical Johnson died last Friday and Mr. Woodward."

Once, while Sgt. George Boylston was firing on attacking Federals, General Beauregard approached him. "Do you know why some shells burst higher than others?" he asked. George picked up two fuses, about the same length. Using his knife, George cut through the fuse covers and showed the general that one was tightly packed with powder while the other was packed loosely. George explained that the loosely packed fuse burns much faster, causing it to explode sooner at a higher level. Beauregard responded, "I think you are right. I will send you some better ones." George reported that the fuses improved after that.

In early 1863, things back in Healing Springs and Blackville were in bad shape. The war had been in progress for almost two years and there were daily reminders of the desperate situation the South faced. Most farmers had grown cotton during the summer of 1861. When they could not sell any of the cotton, they switched to food crops and hay for animals. The Boylstons, the Walkers, the Odoms, the Nevils, and others grew more corn, beans, and wheat, beginning in the summer of 1862. This not only helped them survive, but gave them something to use as barter for other supplies and materials they needed.

161

Part of their crop was shipped by rail to Charleston to support the troops. A half-pound loaf of bread sold for twenty-five cents then, and a barrel of flour cost sixty-five dollars in Charleston.

Some good news arrived in December 1862—newspapers reported the Confederate victory at Fredericksburg, Virginia. General Lee had defeated the Yankees commanded by General Burnside. In January 1863, Burnside tried to outflank Lee but was stopped by Confederate soldiers and the Virginia mud.

In Charleston, the Confederates launched their own naval attack, their gunboats *Chicoro* and *Palmetto State* striking the Federal blockade fleet. The Federals struck back on April 7 when nine Federal ironclads commanded by flag officer Samuel DuPont entered Charleston Harbor and attacked Fort Sumter. Many of the Barnwell District boys were involved in this fight, which drove the Federal ships from the harbor.

Hope was renewed with news of the great Confederate victory at Chancellorsville, Virginia. The victory came at great cost, however—Gen. Stonewall Jackson was mortally wounded.

July 1863 was a month of disasters and the beginning of the end for the Confederacy. Gen. Robert E. Lee was defeated at Gettysburg, Pennsylvania, and Vicksburg, Mississippi, fell to General Grant. The Federals at Charleston began their attacks on Fort Wagner on Morris Island. On July 10, there was an engagement at Willistown Bluff on the Pon Pon (Edisto) River. The first attack on Battery Wagner on Morris Island was repulsed on July 11. A second assault, led by Robert Gould Shaw and the 54th Massachusetts Black Infantry on July 18, produced heavy Federal losses. Twenty-five percent of the attackers perished, including Shaw.

Ellen wrote to George and Pres in January 30, 1863, "I think you all ought to be thankful that you have lost so few of your men. Most every company has lost more than Lamar's Artillery. Sammy left last Thursday not well with the weather being so very bad. When he got to Beauford Bridge he was quite sick. He was fortunate enough to meet with kind friends who took him in their house and nursed him so he was able to ride on Saturday morning. Dr. Brabow ordered him not to go, but to go back home or he would have a severe spell of pneumonia which he had a touch of then. He is almost well now and will go as soon as he can get him a horse since he don't think Clara will hold out. If he can't get one, he thinks of getting a transfer to join another company—he is trying hard to get another horse. Ann and John came over Saturday and remained till Wednesday morning in hopes of meeting Pres. Seems to regret very much not seeing you boys. If she had known you were home Christmas they would certainly have come. . . . Lucian is gone to see Sammy Elkins this evening to find out when he is going down. We will send you meat. If he doesn't get off till it turns cold, we will kill hogs and send some fresh things. I know you will be glad if we can get a cold day to kill. I suppose Cousin Ben Watson has been down to see you all. We are sorry to hear you can't get coffee anymore. We can't sit down and enjoy our coffee anymore when we think of you not having anything to drink. You know our coffee is a substitute, but it does very well. We will parch some and send you some. Annie brought us a box of essence of coffee. It is very nice to mix with wheat. George, it was communion at our church [First Baptist of Blackville] Sunday. How sad it made us feel to look around and see so many vacant seats around the table, seats that were once filled by our friends and loved ones. We pray they might be occupied again by those that were deprived of the privilege of being with us. We pray that we might all meet around the table of the Lord in heaven, if not on earth. Frank Nevils is home quite sick. Thought he would die last week, but he is better now."

During the late summer and fall of 1863, the Federals on Morris Island and those on ship kept up an almost constant bombardment of Fort Sumter. On September 6, the Confederates evacuated Battery Wagner and Morris Island. Fort Sumter and the city of Charleston still held out.

Many young men from the Blackville and Barnwell areas continued to volunteer for service in the Confederate Army in 1863. On September 4, forty-two-year-old Thomas Hightower joined the Boylston brothers in Company I, 5th Regiment, South Carolina Cavalry. The 5th Regiment formed on January 18, 1863, when the 14th cavalry battalion (of which Sam and Lute Boylston were members), the 17th cavalry battalion, and two independent cavalry companies consolidated. Col. Samuel W. Ferguson who initially commanded the regiment was soon replaced by Colonel Dunnovant.

On October 14, 1863, the Confederate submarine *H. L. Hunley* made a practice run near Fort Johnson on James Island. George Boylston, stationed at the fort, went down to the dock to see the "cigar boat." One of the crew members asked George if he wanted to look inside. George climbed down through the small hatch and observed how the submarine was propelled. He wrote that the hand cranks looked like the handles of a railroad handcar. After George climbed out of the *Hunley*, the crew member told him the submarine was going out for a trial run the next morning and if he wanted to see it he should be there early. Anxious to see the vessel in operation, George was on the dock the next morning as the submarine launched. To his surprise the *Hunley* began to sink. He called to the crew member still at the open hatch to get out. The sailor jumped just before the sub sank. Among those who died onboard that day were Horace Hunley, the inventor, and seven crewmen. The sub was later raised. On February 17, 1864, it sank the Federal sloop-of-war *Housatonic*. *Hunley* was the first submarine in naval history to sink a surface vessel. There has been great interest in the *Hunley* since its recovery in 2000.

In February 1864, Presley and George Boylston fought the Federals on James Island as the Yankees on Morris Island were shelling Charleston. George, John C. Williams, and another Barnwell District man under the command of Lieutenant Merritt placed a gun and magazine on the east side of James Island where they could shell the Federals on Morris Island. The Federals paid little attention to Confederate fire until Captain Fleming ordered the rebels to fire solid shot. That got the Feds' attention. They turned their fire away from Charleston and toward the Confederate gun. As George was fusing a shell, the first Federal shot hit their magazine, killing one man and burning two others. The side of George's face was burned, his mustache singed, and his hat blown away. He reported what had happened to Captain Fleming. After the war George received the Confederate Cross of Honor from the United Daughters of the Confederacy. No medals were awarded Confederate soldiers during the Civil War.

In March 1864, Gen. U. S. Grant assumed command of the Union Army. He proceeded to Washington, D. C., and established his headquarters with the Army of the Potomac in Virginia. Immediately he began to build up troops for one final push through Virginia. His target was not Richmond but General Lee's army. Seeing this great buildup of Federal soldiers and supplies, Lee requested that President Davis order all available Confederate soldiers to Virginia. Those cavalrymen protecting the Charleston-Savannah railroad line were ordered to go to Virginia as part of Butler's Brigade, commanded by Gen. M. C. Butler of Edgefield, South Carolina.

Butler's Brigade was composed of the 4th, 5th, and 6th South Carolina Regiments and included cavalrymen from Barnwell County. "That fighting cavalry brigade from South Carolina," as they were known, became one of the most famous Confederate cavalry units of the Civil War. General Butler, who served under Gen. Wade Hampton of General Stuart's command, had his foot shot off by a Yankee artillery shell at the Battle of Brandy Station in June 1863.

Just a short time prior to Lute and Sam Boylston's transferring to Virginia, Lute wrote his father about a skirmish on John's Island:

Adams Run
February 14, 1864

Dear Pa

I take the present opportunity to try to write you a letter. I believe you have seen the news in the papers before this about the little fight on Johns Island but it did not many of our men. We only got 4 or 5 killed and lost 8 prisoners. I believe they were all or near about all of them belonged to the Cadet Rangers. I wrote a letter to Mary on the ninth and just as I got through writing and set it to the P.O., we got orders to saddle up as quick as possible. We did so and then we were all formed in line with the other two companies of cavalry that was here. Then we struck a gallop for Johns Island and it is about 26 or 30 miles from here to where we had to go and we kept the same gate for ten miles. Capt. Wilden commanded the cavalry—we halted then and let our horses walk for about a mile. Then we started in a lope again and never halted until we got to the island. We started from here about 2 o'clock and got there at 4 o'clock. So you may judge how we rode—that was on last Tuesday. The troops on the island had a fight that morning. That was the time they took our prisoners so we put out 8 or 10 pickets that night, but I was not one of them and I was glad. I felt a little tired from riding so far. But the next morning Wednesday we got orders about eight o'clock to saddle up. Then we started and rode our horses about a mile and a half. Then we got orders to dismount and hitch them. We formed in line of skirmishes. We marched on for a mile. We were then in above and a hundred yards from the Yankees. Then they began to fire on the left wing of our company and on the right wing. They kept firing. Then our artillery commenced about the center. Then the Yankees commenced with their artillery and one of the men that was in a company next to us climbed up in a tree to see their movements and the enemy seen him and got the range of us. We all had to lie flat to the ground. We then got orders to fall back. We did so and got to our horses and came back to our camping place. We stayed there that night and most of the next day. General Wise did not attack the Yankees that morning. He was waiting for reinforcements, but the Yankees came up

and attacked our force about 8 o'clock and
just about that time our reinforcements
came up, but we only fought with artillery.
Our cavalry was kept back in reserve. That
was Thursday 11th and the shells fell about
us pretty thick again, but the infantry
and the Yankees began to retreat. Then we
were ordered to go   hitch our horses
    very thick woods right where the
Yankees were fighting. That evening
we were expecting to get right up on the
enemy every minute   told to go on
until we found whether they had left the
island or not. I confess that I felt a little
concern but I put my trust in God, he who
knows all in Heaven and on earth and I
went through safe. We found ten dead
Yankees and ten wounded horses of theirs.
We got down nearly to the end of the island
and Capt. Wilden detailed 12 men to picket
and the rest of us went back to our company
        and next morning we went
skirmishing again but found that they had
all left the island. We came back to our
camping place and stayed there that night
and next morning started back to camp,
that was yesterday, Saturday, got here about
10 o'clock. Tell Sam if he possibly comes
back in 5 to 6 days before his furlough is
out, so I can get to go to see the boys and
come home to see you all for I have a good

deal to tell you all. Tell Sam to be sure and
do so if he can. This leaves me well except
I feel sore from the ride. I must close for the
present. Remember me in your prayers. As
ever your son.

Lucian Boylston

Sam and Lute Boylston and others from Barnwell
District were transported by train with Butler's Brigade
from Charleston to Columbia and then to Petersburg,
Virginia, in May. At Petersburg, the men were ordered to
disembark and assist in the defense of the city. They engaged in battles at Charles Station on May 10, Drewry's
Bluff on May 16, Atkinson's Farm on May 17, and
Charles City Court House on May 24. As their horses
had not arrived, they fought as infantry.

Only a few days later, at Haw's Shop, the 4th and 5th
South Carolina cavalry regiments were engaged in one of
the hardest fought cavalry battles to that time. It was in
this battle that Butler's Brigade earned its reputation as
"that fighting cavalry brigade from South Carolina."

About a week after the Battle of Haw's Shop, Gen.
Wade Hampton's command, which included Butler's Brigade, rode west toward Gordonsville to intercept the Federal cavalry of General Sheridan, sent by Grant to destroy
the railroad. The fight that ensued at Trevilian Station on
June 11 and 12 was one of the bloodiest cavalry battles of
the war. On June 12, Sgt. Sam Boylston, while defending

against repeated Federal assaults, was seriously wounded in the hand. He was taken to the Charlottesville hospital and later to Jackson Hospital in Richmond, where he died on June 20. His wife Lizzie traveled to Richmond by train in January 1865 and brought his body back to Blackville for burial at the First Baptist Church. His grave, along with those of his father, mother, and sisters lie under the present church sanctuary.

Following the battle at Trevilian Station, Lute Boylston spent the next three months fighting with Butler's Brigade around Stony Creek, Virginia, about fifteen miles below Petersburg. He was killed in one of these skirmishes on September 29 and is likely buried at the Sappony Baptist Church near Stony Creek in an unmarked grave.

Three sons of Abraham Odom from Healing Springs fought with Company H of the 17th South Carolina infantry. They saw action in Virginia, North Carolina, and South Carolina, at 2nd Manassas, Antietam, and Five Forks. They also fought at Fort Sumter and Kinston, North Carolina. Two of the young men, Wiatt and Richard, were killed in Virginia, likely at the 2nd Manassas battle in 1862. William J. was the only son serving in the Confederate Army to survive the war. He returned home to Healing Springs after the conflict and lived until 1905.

The Healing Springs Baptist Church and the First Baptist Church of Blackville, as well as other area churches, held regular gatherings of women and young girls to sew homespun garments for local soldiers. Since the majority of able men was away, most small farms were run by grandfathers, women, and young boys.

Throughout the war, churches from all around Blackville routinely sent committees to the local train station to meet scheduled trains transporting wounded and sick soldiers from Charleston to Augusta. These women would walk through the crowded railroad cars distributing food and cool water to the soldiers and offering encouragement. As the war progressed, there was less and less food to distribute.

The situation at home in Healing Springs and Blackville in late 1864 continued to deteriorate. Not only was there a continuous flow of death notices from the battlefront, but many deaths at home from diseases. Also, there was growing concern about General Sherman's capture of Atlanta, Georgia, in September and his march through Georgia with 60,000 troops.

It was hard for the residents of Healing Springs and Blackville to realize that just across the Savannah River in Georgia, about fifty miles away, Sherman foraged property and burned houses. Each day they expected to hear that his troops had crossed the river into South Carolina. They talked of leaving, but since no one knew where Sherman was headed, they decided it was best to stay put. If the Federals did come to Blackville and Healing Springs, they decided, they would hide in the South Edisto River swamp.

The trains continued to arrive in Blackville each day, bringing news of the Federal march through Georgia, southward toward Savannah. Although there was great concern for those in Georgia, there was relief in Blackville and Healing Springs that they would be spared Sherman's wrath. By Christmas, Sherman was in Savannah. It was a sad time for the Boylstons—two sons killed in battle in Virginia, two in harm's way in Charleston, and both Mary and Ellen dead of typhoid fever.

The question of where Sherman would go next was answered in early January 1865 when Federal troops began crossing the Savannah River into South Carolina. It was at this time that Lizzie, Sam Boylston's wife, left Blackville by train on her sad journey to Richmond to bring her husband's body back home for burial. As she returned from Richmond the week of January 5, Sherman began his South Carolina invasion.

As Sherman's left wing crossed the Savannah River at Sister's Ferry just north of Savannah, the train bringing Lizzie and Sam arrived in Blackville. Lizzie sent word to the Boylstons at Oak Grove and the pastor of First Baptist Church from the station. Preparing for Lizzie's return, Austin had dug a fresh grave in the Baptist churchyard beside Sam's sisters Mary and Ellen. Sam's body was promptly buried when Austin, Polly, and other family members and friends arrived. As the service concluded, news arrived that Federals headed toward Branchville and Barnwell. Confederate infantry and cavalry units marched through Blackville toward the Federal advance.

Everyone in Blackville and Healing Springs was in a state of shock. They never dreamed the war would actually come to their homes. Many people loaded their belongings into wagons, trying to move away from Sherman. Most headed west toward Aiken and Augusta. Some chose to remain and protect their homes from Sherman's bummers, but they sent most of their valuables and animals to safe locations. What they did not send away they buried around the farms.

Refugees from Barnwell streamed into Blackville, telling horrifying stories of how Sherman's men burned homes, churches, public buildings, a women's seminary, and the Masonic lodge. Folks in Blackville expected the worst.

As Sherman's troops marched through Barnwell District, they came to the Bell family home where John Bell's wife Cynthia was pregnant, expecting a child at any moment. Soon the bummers were taking all the food and animals including John's only horse. Seeing their horse being led away, John pleaded with the soldiers to leave the horse so his pregnant wife could be carried to the doctor. In an unusual show of kindness, the bummers left the horse.

In the town of Barnwell Sherman's men seem determined to destroy everything in sight. They put many homes and most public buildings to the torch. The flames from the burning buildings could be seen many miles away at night. Most county courthouses in Sherman's path did not survive. However, due to the foresight of Clerk of Court A. V. Eaves, Sheriff Willis W. Woodward, and others all court records including the Winton County Minutes Book had been removed to safety.

By this time there were no more trains arriving from Charleston. The Feds had destroyed the tracks near Branchville. Sherman's four corps, plus General

Kilpatrick's cavalry, marched across South Carolina with little Confederate resistance. On Tuesday, January 7, the first of Kilpatrick's cavalry reached Blackville. There they skirmished with General Wheeler's Confederate cavalry. Federal reconnaissance checked out the Holman and Cannon bridges across the South Edisto River.

As more and more Federal troops poured into Blackville, Kilpatrick's cavalry pushed on toward Williston and White Pond along the railroad route. The Federal troops remaining in Blackville were busy destroying the railroad tracks and plundering. A group of bummers were attacked by Wheeler's cavalry at Holman's Bridge, near the Samuel Reed and Boylston farms. Only Austin and Polly remained in the Boylston house. They kept just enough food to try bribing the bummers not to burn their home. Sherman's troops, however, concentrated on Blackville and caused less damage outside the town.

While ransacking Blackville homes, the bummers' prime target was food for themselves and their horses. If they believed families were hiding food or valuables, they tortured the old men and young boys trying to learn the hiding places. When the Federals reached the Molony home, the old black nanny put a side of meat in a rocking chair on the front porch and sat on it. There she sat rocking one of the Molony babies when the bummers rode up. As usual they took everything they could find. While taking corn from the barn, they dropped some on the ground. After they left, the family picked up the dropped corn. This and the side of meat old nanny sat on was all the food they had left. Picking up dropped corn left by the Federals was an action repeated throughout all of South Carolina as many family histories attest.

Every now and then, a home would be spared. However, those were the exceptions. Most homes and barns in the fifty-mile-wide path of Sherman's troops were burned. Evidence of this could be seen for many years after the war by the lonely chimneys standing like tombstones over the charred remains of burned houses. One home that remained standing was the Shelton home on the Barnwell road. It was believed to have been saved by displaying a Masonic emblem.

Capt. Robert Moore Willis of Williston wrote his wife from Charleston at the time Sherman's men were advancing through South Carolina. He told her how anxious he was about their property and that she should build a lot in some secret place to keep their horses, cattle, and hogs when the enemy is near. As he predicted, Sherman's men arrived at the Willis farm. The Federal cavalrymen, likely Kilpatrick's troops, entered the home and ransacked it. Willis' wife, Susan, was in bed with a new baby when the soldiers arrived. Planning to burn the house, they carried the mother and her baby on the mattress from her bed and placed them on the ground outside. About that time a young Federal officer rode up. Seeing what was happening, he ordered the men to extinguish the fires and return the mother and child to their home. Susan Willis thanked the young officer and asked his name. He responded, "Lt. Walter Tate." She replied, "That will be the name of my baby."

The Federals left Williston and headed toward

Montmorenci and Aiken. At Aiken, Gen. Joe Wheeler's cavalry waited in ambush and drove them back to Montmorenci. From there, Kilpatrick pulled back to White Pond before crossing the South Edisto River at Pine Log Bridge, at present-day Aiken State Park.

While Kilpatrick's cavalry crossed the river, the Federals in Blackville marched out of town toward Guinyard's Bridge, Duncan's Bridge, and Holman's Bridge. Their route toward Duncan's and Holman's Bridges, just east of Jones Island on the South Edisto, led them close to Healing Springs. Having heard of the fresh, cool water at the springs, many of the Federal troops and supply wagons turned off the road and traveled the short distance to Healing Springs. Once there, they filled every container they had with the water.

As it has always done, the spring water soothes friend and foe alike. It is possible that wounded northern bluecoats bathed their wounds in the healing springs as the redcoats had done during the Revolutionary War.

Just south of Duncan's Bridge, the Feds encountered the Boylston homeplace, Oak Grove, while looking for supplies before crossing the South Edisto River. Austin and Polly were standing on the front porch when a Yankee officer and about four of his men on horseback rode into the yard. They stopped under a large oak tree, walked to the front steps, and asked Austin for food and drink. Expecting the Feds would come, Polly had cooked cornbread and ham. The officer said he would come inside to eat, but food must be brought outside for his men. Austin led the officer to the kitchen while Polly prepared four plates of cornbread and fried ham for the men out-side. Placing the plates of food on the edge of the front porch so the men could stand on the ground and eat, Polly returned to join Austin and the officer in the kitchen. Only a few words were exchanged during the meal. While the officer ate, he constantly looked around to make sure there was no one else in the house who might attack him. The Federals departed without doing any harm to the house. However, on their way back to the main road they visited the barn and took the remaining bags of corn and wheat. Austin and Polly felt that was a small price to pay, considering what had happened in Blackville and Barnwell. Likely, the Federals were anxious to be on their way toward Columbia before Wheeler's cav-alry hit their rear guard.

The Samuel Reed home, located close to the route Sherman's men took to Holman's Bridge, was also spared. Elizabeth Boylston Reed, as the legend goes, placed a Bap-tist Church sign in front of the house in hopes Sherman would not burn her home. The church sign was not a complete falsehood since the house was the first meeting place for the First Baptist Church of Blackville. The ploy apparently worked. The house was spared the torch and still stands today, beautifully restored, looking much as it did when Sherman's men marched past.

Word spread throughout the area that Federal troops were preparing to leave Blackville and move north across the South Edisto River. Most of the Federal infantry crossed at Holman's Bridge, while the 20th corps crossed at Duncan's Bridge. Duncan's was a small bridge and not used as much as Holman's and Guinyard's, as this was a wide section of river swamp. The causeways approaching the bridge from the south and north were long and included eleven runs of water that had to be forded. Due to recent heavy rainfall, these fords were about a foot deep. Despite the difficulty, 13,000 Federal soldiers and many wagons crossed the river heading north on Sunday morning, January 1865.

About a mile north of the South Edisto River on high ground stood the Winningham house, built in 1830 with handmade wooden pegs. Federal officers took the house as their headquarters until all their troops had completed crossing the river. Mrs. Winningham was able to save much of her silver and other valuables by placing it in a cabinet and guarding it until the Federals left. Use of the Winningham house by the Federals probably saved it from destruction. This grand old house remained standing until a few years ago.

Prior to the arrival of Federal troops, most South Carolinians living in Sherman's path moved as many of their valuables as possible to the swamps or buried them in remote locations. Wagons loaded with wheat, corn, and dried beans were driven down trails deep into the swamp, along with livestock and crates of chickens. In some cases rafts were loaded with cotton, valuables, and food and floated down the river to an inaccessible area.

Emma Porter Brodie told an interviewer in 1923 how her father, Allen Porter, and brother, Nathan, drove their remaining livestock about thirty miles up the bank of Dean Swamp Creek into Edgefield County. Mrs. Brodie said the Yankees did not discover her clothes placed in a bag and buried in a pig pen or the family china lowered into the nearby mill pond.

About a mile north of the Winningham house, Sherman's bummers entered the yard of the Walker house, which stands about a half mile east of present-day Springfield. This house was built in the early 1830s by a decendent of Nathaniel Walker of Healing Springs. Although most of the food and animals had been removed from the farm before the Federals arrived, the house was not destroyed. At the Walker house some of Sherman's men marched east through Morgantown toward Orangeburg. Others continued toward Columbia.

All communications to the area had stopped when Sherman marched through. Most people only knew what had happened to them or their town. They had no idea of happenings elsewhere. All they knew was that the Yankee storm had come and was now gone away. They needed to put things back in order as well as they could under the circumstances. There were many Barnwell, Blackville, and Healing Springs soldiers still fighting at Charleston and in Virginia. It was not known if they were alive or dead or if they were wounded or captured. All citizens could do was hope and pray for the best. Sherman's men did not destroy the Healing Springs Baptist Church and the First Baptist Church in Blackville. Those who survived Sherman's bummers gathered at the churches to give thanks and to see how they could help each other.

As Sherman entered Columbia on February 17, 1865, Charleston was being evacuated. All able Confederate troops, including Lamar's Artillery, moved by train north-west through Florence toward Cheraw, South Carolina. Included in General Hardee's army were the Boylston brothers, George and Pres. They would continue with Hardee, fighting as infantry in the battles at Aversboro, just north of Fayetteville, North Carolina, and finally at Bentonville, North Carolina, near Goldsboro. The Bentonville battle was the last major battle of the Civil War.

After the Confederates, now under Gen. Joseph E. Johnston, began retreating toward Greensboro, North Carolina, they learned of the surrender of Gen. Robert E. Lee in Virginia. Seeing that further fighting was useless, General Johnston surrendered to General Sherman at Bennett Place, just west of Durham. There were quite a few Confederate soldiers from Barnwell County in North Carolina when Lee's surrender occurred. Among those were George and Pres Boylston and some in their brother Sam's cavalry brigade. Thomas Hightower survived the bloody cavalry battles in Virginia in 1864 and fought Sherman from Columbia, South Carolina, all the way to Hillsboro, North Carolina. He was among the cavalrymen escorting General Johnston to meet General Sherman at Bennett Place.

Most of I Company, 5th South Carolina cavalry regiment, left for home the night before Johnson's surrender and rode about fifty miles south toward the South Carolina line. There they disbanded. The men rode back to their homes in Barnwell County bearing their arms and without surrendering. Had Sam and Lute Boylston survived the 1864 Virginia battles, they would have been with these men. Infantrymen also left early. An officer approached George and Pres informing them of the next day's events. He said he and others were not willing to surrender and were leaving that night for home. George and Pres agreed to leave with them. The soldiers began their long walk from North Carolina, near Greensboro, to Blackville, a distance of about 250 miles. Capt. Robert Moore Willis of Williston was in the hospital in Greensboro when Johnston surrendered and unable to accompany the Barnwell County soldiers.

With the terrible war finally over, thousands of Confederate soldiers began making their way back to South Carolina, most of them on foot. For some, it would take months to reach home. During that time, their families waited, not knowing if they were alive or dead. For George and Pres it took only about a month to reach Healing Springs. At night they slept in barns and asked for food from homes along the way. It was March and the weather was still cold. Many days it rained. Some of the men who survived the war now became ill on their walk home and died on the journey.

As Austin and Polly were home praying for the protection of their sons and hoping they were alive, they were trying to put their lives back in order. Spring was approaching and the fields had to be prepared. Each day about sunrise Austin hitched up his only mule, which had been hidden in the swamp, to his plow and began preparing his fields for planting. He had saved one bushel of seed corn and a bushel of wheat. These would be the beginning of his recovery. There was no thought of making a profit. What was needed now was food! He would earn profits later to pay his taxes. Austin and Polly found themselves where their parents and grandparents had been seventy-five years earlier—starting from scratch. Fortunately, Austin inherited a stubborn streak and determined to rebuild his farm. After about a month he had his fields ready and he was beginning to plant.

One can imagine how it was when George and Pres Boylston came home from the war: Late one afternoon in mid-April, a beautiful spring day, Austin's hunting dogs began to bark. He had just come in from the fields and was putting the mule in the lot. Polly was cooking supper. As Austin walked to the edge of the lot, he saw the dogs run by, headed for the main road. Looking after them, toward the river, he could see two figures coming up the road. To his surprise the dogs ran right up to the men without barking. Austin felt a charge of electricity run through his body. The two walking toward the house, he thought, just might be George and Pres. He called to Polly to come quick. Once she reached the front porch and took one look down the road, her instinct as a mother told her that her sons were home. She turned her eyes upward and thanked God for protecting her boys. As Polly descended the front steps, Austin ran down the road. Austin was generally a reserved person and showed little emotion. However, the joy of seeing his lost sons overcame him as he rushed to greet George and Pres. Austin hugged and kissed his boys lifting each completely off the ground with his embrace. About the time he put George down and was hugging Pres, Polly reached them, tears streaming down her face. George gave her a big hug and a kiss, lifting her feet off the ground and swinging her around. As soon as he put her down, Pres grabbed her for more kisses and hugs.

Arms around each other, they slowly walked up the road toward the old homeplace, while the dogs ran around them, barking. The great joy in the Boylston family was dulled by the sadness for Sam and Lute who did not survive the war. Also, the brothers cried over the loss of their loving sisters, Mary and Ellen, who had written letters so faithfully during the war only to die of typhoid fever before their return.

The reunion of the Boylstons was one of hundreds of such reunions in Barnwell District following the Civil War. Each family had its own special joy and sorrow. Hardly a family was spared heartache. After the initial happy homecoming and some food and rest, returning soldiers who were able immediately set to work on the farms to make sure families had enough food for the next winter.

George and Pres took over most of the heavy work Austin had been doing. Soon, life was settling back to normal and it appeared they would make it. The next Sunday, the Boylstons, along with other returned veterans, began to fill the pews again at the Healing Springs and Blackville Baptist churches.

One of the Confederate's most famous officers was Brig. Gen. Johnson Hagood, born in Barnwell County on February 21, 1829. Hagood graduated from the South

Carolina Military Academy (The Citadel) in 1847. He studied law and was admitted to the bar in 1850. When South Carolina seceded, he held the rank of brigadier general. Hagood was appointed colonel of the 1st South Carolina infantry regiment and participated in the bombardment of Fort Sumter. In June 1861, he moved to Virginia and fought in the battle of First Manassas. He and his regiment returned to South Carolina and fought in the Secessionville battle in June 1862. After Secessionville, Hagood was promoted to brigadier general. He fought in the Morris Island battles, and in May 1864 returned to Virginia with part of his brigade and fought near Petersburg and at Cold Harbor. In August 1864 he and his men defended the Weldon Railroad. In December 1864 Hagood moved to Wilmington, North Carolina, to defend Fort Fisher. In 1865 he fought in the battles at Kinston and Bentonville. He surrendered at Bennett Place near Durham. Hagood married Eloise Butler, daughter of Sen. A. P. Butler, Gen. M. C. Butler's uncle. General Hagood died in Barnwell on January 4, 1898.

Lt. Francis Marion Bamberg, a native of Barnwell District (in a section now part of Bamberg County), served with distinction during the war. He enlisted in 1861 as a private in Hart's battery of light artillery in Hampton's Legion. In 1862 he was appointed first lieutenant. He fought under Generals Hart, Stuart, Hampton, and Butler during some of the fiercest battles of the Civil War. Although his battery was under Federal fire 142 times, Bamberg was not wounded. He surrendered in 1865 at Greensboro, North Carolina. After the war he returned to Barnwell County and entered the mercantile business in Bamberg.

Frank Henry Creech of Allendale enlisted in 1861 as a private in Company C, Johnson Hagood's infantry regiment. He was disabled by a wound to his lung at Fort Harrison in 1864. In 1878 he was elected county commissioner of Barnwell County and in 1880, sheriff.

Robert Aldrich, the second son of Judge A. P. Aldrich of Barnwell District, was born at The Oaks, his parents' homeplace in 1844. He was a South Carolina Military Academy cadet in 1861. In 1862 he became a part of the 6th South Carolina cavalry regiment known as the cadet regiment. He was promoted to the regiment adjutant and in 1864 commanded a battalion of dismounted cavalry in the Virginia campaigns. In late 1864 Aldrich was promoted to assistant inspector general of Maj. Gen. P. M. B. Young's brigade and served in that capacity until the end of the war. Young's Brigade and Butler's Brigade fought in most of the same battles. In 1876, Aldrich was elected to the legislature from Barnwell County.

Lieutenant Richard Best, a native of Barnwell County, enlisted as a private in Company E of Hagood's 1st South Carolina infantry regiment. Over the next few months he was promoted to corporal, sergeant, and second lieutenant. After the battle of Second Manassas on August 30, 1862, he was promoted to first lieutenant. He fought with Hagood's regiment in most major battles in Virginia. He was severely wounded at the battle of Sharpsburg in 1862 and again in 1864. He married Clio Legard Bignon of Barnwell in 1862.

Jacob David Felder, born in 1844 near Bamberg in Barnwell County, enlisted in 1861 as a private in Company H of Hampton's Legion. During the last year of the war he was made color guard. He had the distinction of being the last Confederate in Virginia to kill a Federal soldier, having shot Col. J. R. Root of the 15th New York cavalry the night before General Lee surrendered. Felder encountered a body of horsemen and thought they were Confederates. When he called to them, Colonel Root fired a pistol at him. Felder then shot Root, killing him instantly. Felder surrendered at Appomattox. In 1866, he married Mary E. Cox of Bamberg.

Lieutenant Richard Creech Roberts of Barnwell County enlisted in Hagood's 1st South Carolina infantry regiment as first sergeant. Later he became a private in Company D, 3rd South Carolina cavalry. Soon after, he was promoted to second lieutenant. He fought against Sherman during his march through the Carolinas. After the war he returned to Barnwell County and resumed his dentistry practice. He married Sarah E. Dunn of Barnwell County in 1860.

Barnwell County native Josiah Dickinson was born near Bamberg. He attended the Arsenal, a Columbia military school, and was operating a store at Buford's Bridge in 1861. He entered Confederate service in the spring of 1862 as a lieutenant in Company G, 17th South Carolina infantry and fought in many Virginia and North Carolina battles. When the war ended, he returned to Buford's Bridge. He was the first county treasurer for Bamberg County. His wife was Eugenia W. Maye of Barnwell

County.

Patrick William Farrell, a native of Ireland, came with his parents to America in 1850. He attended school in Barnwell County and in 1860 moved to Charleston. When the war began he joined Captain Chichester's company of Zouave cadets at Castle Pinckney as a private. In 1862 he joined Walter's battery, Washington light artillery. After the war he moved to Blackville where he opened Farrell's store. In 1870, he married Mrs. Caroline Columbia (Rush) Sanders, a widow from Barnwell County. His daughter Anna married John O'Gorman of Blackville.

It is interesting to note that during the entire Civil War the official minutes of the Healing Springs Baptist Church never mentioned the conflict in any respect. It had to be a conscious decision by the church, considering the suffering and number of deaths in their membership. The only period where there are no church minutes is during February and March 1865 when Sherman's troops were marching through Blackville and Healing Springs.

RECONSTRUCTION

The main focus of life among farmers around Healing Springs and Blackville after the Civil War was survival. They had reached rock bottom. There was truly nowhere to go but up. For the most part, the farmers stayed on their farms and avoided contact with others, except at church. There was little concern about local, county, state or national government. However, those who were in leadership roles prior to the war, such as large farmers and plantation owners, tried to resume those roles when the war was over.

By June 1865, most black Carolinians knew they were free from slavery. Some former slaveowners told them about their freedom. Others did not learn they were free until Federal soldiers riding through the countryside told them. Former slaves, realizing they were free to do what they pleased, reacted in different ways. Most blacks in Barnwell District decided to continue on the farms they had worked as slaves. Some worked for wages, others as sharecroppers.

Most former slaves who left the farms formed their own neighborhoods in the towns and villages. They chose to live in segregated areas, away from the whites. These individuals hired themselves out as temporary farm labor. Some of the large farmers in the area conspired to keep wages low for black laborers.

Sharecropping was the most common system of employing blacks on farms. In return for planting and harvesting crops, black sharecroppers were given about one-third of the cotton produced. Some were also given a plot of land to farm for themselves, usually about fifty acres.

Many whites feared a black uprising. For over one hundred years the slaveowners had used the threat of a slave uprising to gain support for slavery by whites who did not own slaves. Now that black Carolinians, who outnumbered whites, were free to do as they pleased, some whites expected the worst. Their fears never materialized. For the most part, former slaves accepted their freedom and went on with their lives. There were very few incidents of retaliation. The primary concern of blacks was the same as white farmers—to provide for their families.

Former slaves around Healing Springs and Blackville were encouraged to join the local white churches. Both the Healing Springs and Blackville Baptist churches had many black members. Once the war was over and slaves were free, the Baptist and Methodist churches tried to keep their black members. Only a few stayed, however. One freed slave remained at the Healing Springs Baptist Church until 1920. Most black Baptists decided to form their own church.

In 1866 black members of the Healing Springs Baptist Church and other local churches established the first all black Baptist church in Blackville. Rev. James Tolbert of Augusta organized the Macedonia Baptist Church. Over time this church helped found seven other black congregations and the Macedonia Association. The Macedonia Church also established its own school, which operated until public education was offered.

The provisional governor of South Carolina, Benjamin Franklin Perry, called a constitutional convention in Columbia in September 1865. One act of the convention was to acknowledge that slaves in South Carolina were free. Alfred P. Aldrich of the Barnwell District voted "no" to this acknowledgement.

Initially, there was general integration of black and white Carolinians throughout the state in public places and in government. Some blacks and whites tried to work together to move the state forward. However, there would be little harmony as the Republicans pressed through their own form of reconstruction. In March 1867, the Federal Republican government dissolved the initial state governments in the South and established five military districts.

One of the successes of the South Carolina reconstruction assembly was the establishment of tax-supported public education for blacks and whites.

In 1868, the boundaries of Barnwell County changed. A portion of it formed the new Aiken County.

Most South Carolina farmers, including those around Healing Springs and Blackville, were having a hard time making enough money to pay the taxes on their farms. Initially, they grew only the food needed for survival. Over the next few years, some money crops such as cotton began to be sold for profit. The fortunate farmers sold just enough to cover their taxes. Many did not. In 1873 about 270,000 acres of land was seized for failure to pay taxes. One year later the number of acres seized increased to 400,000.

Once George William and Presley Jefferson Boylston helped their father Austin put his farm back in order, they both married local Blackville women. George married Fannie F. Crum on February 17, 1866, and Presley married Fannie's sister, Mary Crum Moorer, a widow, about the same time. Both George and Presley were farmers like their dad and began establishing homes and families of their own.

George's wife Fannie died on August 16, 1867. The following November 25, 1868, he married Carrie Riley. They had five children over the next eight years. They also adopted a child September 1, 1884. Their oldest son Belton would attend medical school in Baltimore, Maryland. All of their children attended colleges or educational institutes.

Presley and Mary had ten children—six boys and four girls. Their descendants would spread over the years through Georgia and Florida. Family reunions are still held in Savannah, Georgia.

Both George and Presley remained active in the First Baptist Church of Blackville, which their father Austin helped establish. George was a deacon in the church and served for sixteen years on the executive committee of the Barnwell Baptist Association. He also served as a Blackville school trustee in 1876.

George Boylston's records show purchases made, typical for residents of Healing Springs and Blackville at the time: from the Farrell & Co. store in Blackville in 1870, a bottle of turpentine for 40¢, four pounds of cheese for $1, and one-half gallon of whiskey for $2.05. Local purchases in 1873 included twenty yards of print cloth for $3, one pair of silk gloves for 15¢, one ounce of gum camphor for 15¢, one gallon of molasses for 50¢, and one milk pail for 15¢.

A letter to George from his brother-in-law in 1879 described life on the farm.

Caw Caw Hills
March 17, 1879

Dear George:
I have been driven indoors by rain. I was putting down acid and cottonseed
for cotton. And I am obliged to go to town in a day or two. Therefore, I will make use of the time in sending you a few lines. I am very much obliged to you for sending the seed corn. I am proud of it although I have some brag corn seed that I have not tested yet to my satisfaction that of Vastine. The Hodges corn (old gourd seed) I lay aside. I do not like it at all. It takes too long to get out corn for grits too soft entirely. I like the looks of your corn. I think it is all right. Vastine's seed is very good. The fault I have of that   it takes too long to make, about 2 weeks behind ordinary corn. I have not planted any corn yet. I will begin on the 20th, I think. My corn land was prepared sometime ago, but instead of planting I went to putting down cottonseed and acid. I put

ten to twelve bushels per acre and 130 to 150 lbs. of acid phosphate. I can plant my corn in three days if I get a good run on it. Garden very backward. Mollie planted seeds early enough, but on account of dry weather

did not get a good stand. Those that came look badly. I think I will be ready to plant cotton early, if the weather is favorable. I will plant a little sooner than usual. I have traded my old Barton planter to Uncle   for one of West's guano distributors. I have been putting down guano with it and I tell you it lacks right good deal of being a humbug. I have bought a   planter   cost me freight included $4.35. We are tolerably well at present. Mollie had a severe splitting headache Saturday. I hope mother's stay with you will improve her. For several weeks she has had the headaches nearly all the time, just before she went over. Julia Stack has a fine boy. So has Nealy Robinson

ten days apart. The grip or coughs and cold have abated to a great extent. Well George, I will close for this time, my news box is getting about as empty as a contribution box and in fact I am a little tired and cramps besides so I beg to be excused for this evening. Write soon and tell me how tall your corn is.

Your Brother (in-law)
Rhett Riley

Apparently, George was successful in his planting. In 1890 he purchased a cotton gin from the Brown Cotton Gin Company in New London, Connecticut, for about $200. It cost him $14.80 to ship the gin by railroad. His cotton ginning business was good. Records show he ginned 400 standard square 500-pound bales of cotton in 1900.

News reached Blackville of serious problems in state government in Columbia. What was happening would affect state citizens for many years into the future. Under Reconstruction governors Scott and Moses state government was filled with graft and corruption from 1872 to 1874. They issued twice as many state bonds as authorized by the General Assembly. It would take until 1946 for South Carolina to finally pay off this debt.

Freed black Carolinians were able to purchase their own farms with help from the South Carolina Land Commission. The Commission purchased land between 1869 and 1877 and sold it to small farmers, most of whom were blacks. Some of these farms are still owned by descendants of the original black owners.

Unlike what happened at the end of World War II, when the United States made a major commitment to help our enemies Germany and Japan recover rapidly, there was no similar commitment by the Washington Republicans. On the contrary, the Federal government did all they could to punish the South. They established the Freeman's Bureau, which was designed, as the name implies, to assist freed black slaves. This organization helped many blacks and a few whites. The whites who were helped were those starving with no way to get food. At this time, the United States (because of industry in the North) was one of the greatest industrial powers on earth.

Austin Boylston and other Barnwell County farmers were having a rough time. They were not able to farm all their land. Most of the crops they did raise could not be sold, due to a lack of buyers. Just about the time things began looking up for the farmers, the national depression of 1873 hit and interest rates grew to around twenty-five percent. Those who could, held on, hoping things would soon improve. Over the first few years after the war ended, there was a gradual withdrawal of Federal troops from South Carolina. By 1868, there were only 881 Federal troops left in the state. Seldom were any Federal troops seen in Blackville and those few were usually riding the train.

In the late 1860s, white organizations such as the Ku Klux Klan (KKK) formed and became militant against the South Carolina Reconstruction government. Many government officials and supporters of Reconstruction were attacked. In response to these attacks on state officials, a new state militia was created to protect black Carolinians, especially black government officials. Before the end of 1870, there were 100,000 militiamen, mostly black. There was a fear of open conflict between the militiamen and the KKK. In response to this threat, the Federal government sent more troops into South Carolina.

News of these attacks and confrontations arrived in Blackville and Healing Springs from Columbia and Charleston, but most local citizens paid little attention. They were too busy trying to rebuild their farms and their lives after the war. Rich farmers were still involved in politics, of course, and wanted to regain control of state government. The small farmer, however, had seen enough armed conflict and wanted only to be left alone.

When former Confederate general Wade Hampton became involved in South Carolina politics in 1872, the mood of the general public, including folks from Barnwell County, changed. Hampton was the most respected South Carolina Confederate general. There were thousands of former Confederate cavalrymen, including those from Barnwell and Edgefield Counties, who served under Generals Hampton and M. C. Butler. They were loyal and devoted followers during the war and would continue following their former superiors in recapturing their state from the radical Republicans.

Once the former Confederate soldiers entered the South Carolina political arena, the whole campaign changed. Hampton supporters, mostly former Confederates, began to organize political action groups called clubs. One of the clubs was the Allendale Rifle Club. These clubs marched to political activist meetings, disrupting them. There is no question the clubs were a source of political power, through militant force. They were determined to return the Democrats to power.

About this time, there was a riot in Hamburg, South Carolina, which terminated the Charleston-Hamburg railroad. Based on accounts, a black militia company had blocked the street so a white resident of North Augusta could not get to his home. This led to a confrontation where a number of blacks were killed. This riot received extensive publicity across the state and nation and was followed by an armed confrontation between blacks and whites in the town of Ellenton, South Carolina.

The Federal government's response to the attacks in South Carolina was to increase their military presence and order the "rifle clubs" to disband. By then, the tide had changed and the support for Hampton in South Carolina was overwhelming. There was growing concern about the Federal Republican administration across the nation. The national Democrats wanted to resume control of the Federal government and saw the southern Democrats as a way to achieve a majority. Hampton supporters in South Carolina had support nationally. Knowing they had this support, the state's political clubs continued to operate. In most cases they only changed their names. The Allendale Rifle Club became the Allendale Mounted Baseball Team. Former Confederate generals Hampton, Butler, and M. W. Gary, along with hundreds of their supporters rode throughout the state, speaking to crowds and shaking hands. People came from miles around to see Hampton and urge him on. The procession was like a mounted cavalry brigade.

In the election of 1876, Hampton won with 92,261 votes to Chamberlain's 91,127 votes. It was not strictly a black and white division of voters. Hampton won the election with 17,000 black votes. Following the election, all Federal troops were pulled out of South Carolina. Since the election was contested, there were two state governments trying to operate in South Carolina. Finally Hampton's Democrats won out and assumed power. This was the beginning of the end of Reconstruction in South

Carolina. There was a sigh of relief by most citizens, both black and white. They were ready for conflict to cease. Hampton initially tried to involve black Carolinians in state government. He appointed 86 blacks to state offices. The blacks were encouraged by this show of cooperation.

During Reconstruction, in 1869, the seat of Barnwell County government had moved from Barnwell to Blackville. The court was temporarily housed in a church until the new courthouse was built in 1871 at a cost of $8,000. In 1874 there was a county referendum concerning the permanent location of the county seat. The fact that Blackville had a major railroad was an important factor. In 1875, popular vote returned the county seat to Barnwell. This was an important turn of events for both towns, since in the long run Barnwell would benefit from the location of the court, and state and county services. In contrast, Blackville would slowly decline. For many years, though—until the 1930s—Blackville continued to prosper from agriculture and the railroad.

The *Peoples Newspaper* of Barnwell usually covered international, national, state, and local news in the 1870s. Those reading the paper were well informed of most current events. Most editions included a column specifically about Blackville and Healing Springs. These articles contained local trivia and gossip. Usually, events were described without giving names, causing people to debate the identity of the person alluded to. Because of the turbulent 1870s, most articles had a political bent.

A headline in the *Peoples Newspaper* dated October 25, 1887, announced, "Days Doings in Blackville." The article read, "The town was very lively on Saturday. There was a large trade in both cotton and corn. There was a dance and a social at the residence of Mr. Mike Brown on Monday night. The moon was full; the sky clear, making the evening very inviting. There was quite a large assemblage of the fair ones of our town and enough young gentlemen to 'pair off' as they say in Congress."

During Reconstruction, the *Peoples Newspaper* reported on numerous paramilitary organizations, known as rifle clubs. Two of these were the Gordon Volunteers and the Edisto Grays. These groups held meetings, parades, and picnics, often attended by a hundred or more people.

One long article on September 18, 1878, sported the headline "Hampton and Home Rule in the Banner County." The article described the magnificent ovation for the Red Shirts of Barnwell County who supported Hampton.

An interesting article appeared in the February 27, 1879, edition, which read, "G. H. Hope, Esq., General Agent of the Singer Sewing Machine Company located in Charleston, SC paid this town [Blackville] a visit last week." This clearly shows the interest in the sewing machine as a new invention that revolutionized the making of clothes in homes.

Healing Springs Baptist Church was still the focal point of the community throughout the 1870s. The first Sunday school organizational meeting was held on May 27, 1880, and most of the news in the local newspaper was about church meetings. Healing Springs Academy, located between the church and the springs, still operated.

READJUSTMENT

Reconstruction ended in 1877 when newly elected President Rutherford B. Hayes, a Republican, withdrew Federal troops from the South. Between that time and 1900 there was a period of readjustment in South Carolina and the rest of the South. The Federal troop removal was to pacify the South after Hayes won a contested election over Samuel J. Tilden. A congressional commission awarded the election to Hayes.

The North was enjoying "the Gilded Age," so-called by Mark Twain. Americans were on the move to large cities and the West. Northern industry, which flourished during the Civil War, now expanded greatly. People entered the northern factories from southern farms and the income of average northern workers increased. However, this wage increase was small compared to the great profits of factory owners.

It was during this "Gilded Age" the term "poor folks down South" originated. In general this was an accurate term, because there was no comparison between the standards of living of northerners and southerners. They were at opposite ends of the economic scale. Little, if anything, was being done by the Federal government to improve the situation in the South.

As northern big business was becoming even bigger, taking advantage of the vast American resources in petroleum, iron ore, copper, and coal, southern farmers were beginning to organize. The National Grange had formed in 1867 and farmer's alliances and cooperatives were gaining popularity in the 1880s. Most of these alliances were an effort to break the railroad monopoly and reduce charges for shipping farm products. Farmer concerns led to the enactment in 1887 of the Interstate Commerce Act.

Although attendance at public schools increased greatly after the Civil War, illiteracy in the South was high. Efforts were made to improve schools around Healing Springs and Blackville, but progress was slow. Many schools were still one-room buildings.

Again, just as things were looking up, disaster struck. J. Reid Boylston of Allendale, a distant cousin of the Blackville Boylstons, whose ancestors had come from England to New England, back to England, and then to Charleston in 1794, described the Charleston earthquake of 1886 in an August 30, 1936, *News and Courier* article. Reid was the mail agent on the last of the summer excursion trains from the mountains to the coast. His train pulled out of Columbia about 4:30 P.M. on its way to Charleston. Before the train reached Charleston the great earthquake of August 31, 1886, struck. The first indication that something was wrong was the train's sudden stop. When the express messenger was asked, "What's wrong?" he responded, "Earthquake!" The train shook from a second, more severe shock. Following the second shock wave, the train moved slowly ahead in the darkness. People standing along the tracks were crying and shouting that judgment day had come. At Summerville, Mr. Averil, the railroad superintendent, shouted, "For God's sake, stop!"

It was good they did, since the track rails ahead were bent into an "S" shape. One of these rails was later sent to the Smithsonian Institute in Washington. A sidetrack was located for the continued ride to Charleston after staying the night in Summerville. The next afternoon, September 1, as they waited in Summerville, another aftershock shook Reid off the track he was sitting on.

Proceeding slowly, the train arrived in Charleston about dark on September 1. The train on which Reid rode was the first to enter the city after the earthquake. A local newspaper quoted Reid: "At the northwest corner of Smith and Calhoun streets was my father's home. His garden was filled with tents of those afraid to stay indoors. On that one lot six babies were born during the 12 hours after the first shock. All the food in our house had gone to those families camping in our yard. Debris covered the ground. There were large cracks in the streets. There was no food. The livestock raised a clamor at each aftershock." During the next few days, Reid Boylston would make several train trips between Charleston and Allendale, taking food and relief to those in the damaged city.

The great Charleston earthquake, measuring 6.6 on the Richter scale, was felt all over South Carolina. One of George Boylston's cousins, Charlie Boylston, lived near Salley, South Carolina, at the time of the earthquake. Everyone was afraid their houses would fall on them, so when they felt an aftershock they rushed outside as fast as they could. Charlie decided to jump out the window, which was about ten feet off the ground. He threw up the sash and jumped. He failed, however, to move fast enough. The window came flying back down, catching his long nightshirt. Once the shock was over, everyone began calling to each other to ensure that all were safe. Cousin Charlie was not among them. Finally, they heard someone hollering at the side of the house. There, they saw Charlie hanging by his nightshirt, naked as a jaybird. Everyone had a big laugh, except Charlie. He knew the family would remember the event forever—and it has!

By 1887, Blackville had about rebuilt after the destruction of Sherman's troops in February 1865 and the town was growing rapidly with many new businesses. On March 16, 1887, disaster struck in the form of a firestorm, which swept through the town. About eighty white and forty-five black people were made homeless and fifty-seven buildings burned to the ground. The fire was first seen on the roof of P. W. Farrell's store about 1:15 A.M., started perhaps by a spark from a passing train. The flames spread by the wind to other structures. As the fire burned, people carried goods from the stores along Railroad Avenue. Sparks fell on the goods, destroying them anyway. A call for help brought the Aiken Fire Company, about 30 miles away, in a train at fifty miles per hour. The firefighters helped bring the fire under control. In the end, about thirteen acres burned. Some of the burned businesses included Simon Brown's, P. W. Farrell's, W. J. Martin & Son, Still Brothers, and Martin Keeler's.

Blackville citizens opened their doors to the fire victims. Neighboring towns sent aid including food and clothes. As they did after Sherman's visit, the citizens of Blackville, with the help of neighboring communities, began rebuilding. This time they built with brick.

There were about four times more farms in the late 1890s as there were in 1860. By 1895, Healing Springs and Blackville farmers were raising twice as much cotton as before the war, but the cotton price was too low for the farmers to make much profit. About this time, North and South Carolina began to benefit from northern labor unrest and increasing wages. Some of the northern textile mill owners began to build mills in the South. Indirectly, this would help most South Carolina farmers. There was an increase in tobacco production in North Carolina and Virginia, and some South Carolina farmers began to grow tobacco as a high-income crop.

To most people living in the North, the 1890s were known as the "Gay Nineties." Such was not the case for most Southerners, like those living around Healing Springs and Blackville. Things were better, but a long way from being gay. The average pay was $12 a week for sixty hours work. Milk cost 6¢ per quart and steak 12¢ per pound. These prices seem low by today's standards, but they were high for those having little money.

One thing that did begin to appear in the South, as well as the North, during the Victorian Era was more freedom for women. Maybe it was the freeing of the slaves that made women realize that in some respects they were treated like slaves. As living conditions improved, Southern women, who had always been strong in church and at home, began to assert themselves. They wanted equal treatment under the law and in the community. This movement would continue for over 100 years—and continues today. Women began to attend college, and many female colleges were established in South Carolina. Women's clothes also changed in the 1890s when Charles Dana Gibson's "Gibson Girl" free styles became popular. New magazines were established, which appealed to more liberated women—*Cosmopolitan, Ladies Home Journal,* and *Good Housekeeping.* Work at home also improved during the 1880s and 1890s. Since the Singer sewing machine was about half the cost it had been, almost every home had a sewing machine. Much less time was required to sew clothes, giving women more leisure time. Now, they could enjoy music on one of Thomas Edison's hand-cranked phonographs. The favorite song was "Carry Me Back to Old Virginny."

Those living in the Healing Springs community and in Blackville were enjoying the many new inventions and products of the period, including the telephone, photography, Ivory soap, and electric lights. Now, Chase and Sanborn's roasted coffee could be purchased in cans.

The railroad had come to the Healing Springs community around 1887 when the Blackville-Alston-Newberry Railroad was completed to the kaolin mines in Aiken County. At that time Walker Station obtained its designation.

Improved farm machinery made farms less labor intensive. A McCormick reaper, a big advance in harvesting, could be bought for about $1,500. Cream was now separated from milk by centrifugal separators. The need for less manual labor and the increasing "Jim Crow" segregation laws caused many blacks to leave South Carolina. On the surface there were no visible racial problems in Blackville and the Healing Springs area. Older blacks realized there was little they could do to change the situation in the South and did not discourage their older children from moving to the North and West where they would have more opportunity and their civil rights would be better protected. Many young black adults with drive and initiative to improve racial conditions of the South were forced to leave. Seventy-five years passed before descendants of this generation began returning to their southern roots.

The 1890s brought changes across the United States. Internal gasoline combustion engines began to impact the development of motorcars and farm tractors. By the late 1940s, the use of mules in farming would be almost extinct. Railroads were also going through changes. In 1894, the Southern Railway System organized and connecting tracks were built to most parts of the state.

By the late 1890s, there was a growing interest in bottled mineral water and soda pop (soft drinks). Coca-Cola, Pepsi-Cola, and Dr. Pepper were now being sold along with ginger ale, sarsaparilla, and root beer. White Rock Mineral Water was distributed widely. There was talk about the possibility of bottling Healing Springs Mineral Water.

Post-Civil War politicians replaced the old Civil War veterans, who were active in ending Reconstruction. Tillmanites gained control of South Carolina politics when Benjamin R. Tillman was elected governor in 1890. The Tillmanites included most of the farmers around

Healing Springs and Blackville who believed Tillman would help them increase their farm profits. Soon after his election, Tillman rewrote the state constitution and all but eliminated voting rights of blacks. In 1895, Tillman became a U. S. Senator, defeating former Confederate general M. C. Butler of Edgefield.

Most of the nation, especially people in the South had no desire for more war. They had seen enough fighting during the Civil War to last a lifetime. As often happens though, the generation coming of age after the war heard only the glory of war—not the pain and suffering. They looked forward to the opportunity of following their fathers, grandfathers, and uncles into battle. Their chance came in 1898 with the Spanish-American War. Spain, which ruled Cuba, sent about 200,000 troops to the island in 1895 to crush a revolt. Three years later, the conflict still not resolved, the United States sent the battleship *Maine* to Havana Harbor as a show of strength. On the night of February 15, 1898, there was an explosion on the *Maine* and the ship sank with 260 sailors onboard. On April 21, 1898, the United States declared war on Spain. This war greatly expanded U. S. territory and resulted in the country becoming a world power.

THE NEW CENTURY

In 1899, as the twentieth century approached, citizens of Healing Springs and Blackville looked back with pride at the community's accomplishments over the preceding 100 years. They knew how hard their grandparents had worked to build homes in the wilderness and how heroically their parents struggled during the Civil War and Reconstruction. Now, their generation was preparing to meet the challenges of a new century. America was not the same as it had been before the great war. There was no longer a western frontier. Technology had brought the country into a new age and new inventions were introduced monthly. Americans searched for greater opportunities.

Between 1890 and 1910 over thirteen million immigrated to the United States. Most of the new immigrants went to large northern cities to work in the factories. It was reported during this period that in one New England textile mill alone twenty-five different languages were spoken. Where the country's early European settlers had been white—Anglo-Saxon and Protestant—the nation was now filling with white, black, and yellow.

Rural America—areas such as Healing Springs and Blackville—was not changing as rapidly as the more populated sections of the nation. This was especially true in the South where people still struggled to rebuild lives demolished during the Civil War. Healing Springs and Blackville remained to a large degree places of innocence—quiet refuges, with dirt roads and horse-drawn carriages. Baptist churches were still the focal points of community activity and social life. People still used kerosene lamps and outhouses. Women wore tight corsets.

The suffrage movement was underway. Women began to express themselves more concerning their rights. Men—and some women—believed that giving women the right to vote was dangerous for women and would undermine the family. Feminist Carrie Chapman Catt wrote, "American women who know the history of their country, will always resent the fact that American men chose to enfranchise Negroes fresh from slavery before enhancing their wives and mothers." Most southern women had experienced much equality in helping build their new homes in the wilderness. They worked side by side with their husbands in the fields and were involved in making major decisions. Most women looked on the suffrage movement as a logical step in the country's development.

Queen Victoria died in January 1900 after a reign of sixty-four years. England would never be the same again. That same year President McKinley was assassinated and Theodore Roosevelt became the youngest president of the United States at age forty-two. The life expectancy for white males born in America in 1901 was forty-eight years—fifty-one years for white females. Many diseases had become better controlled, but hookworm was still widespread throughout South Carolina. Songs of the times included "In the Good Old Summertime," "Bill Bailey, Won't You Please Come Home," "In the Sweet By and

By," and "I Love You Truly."

When Ben Tillman became governor of South Carolina, quality of life deteriorated for black Carolinians. Separate black and white schools were mandated; only tax-paying, literate voters could serve as jurors, thus, eliminating most blacks; and there were "whites only" and "coloreds only" signs everywhere in public places. Blacks were to shop in town only on Saturdays in some rural towns, and they were expected to enter white people's houses by the back door.

Railroads continued to bring growth and increased wealth for communities. Now, more and more emphasis was placed on encouraging the establishment of textile mills, especially in the Upstate. Northern mills continued to move south to take advantage of low labor costs and lack of union activity. It was during the early 1900s that child labor laws were passed to prohibit children under ten years of age from working in factories, mines, or mills. By 1905, this age had been increased to twelve.

Healing Springs and Blackville worked to improve living conditions for all its citizens. Schools for blacks and whites were upgraded, libraries were built, and parks were created.

A survey in 1910 revealed that only thirteen proper high schools existed in South Carolina, including one in Bamberg. Improved education was not only needed in South Carolina but throughout the nation, since the average American adult of that era had only five years of schooling. In 1878, when there was an increased emphasis on providing opportunities for education, a two-story boarding school had been built on the east side of the road leading to Healing Springs from Highway 3, just south of Healing Springs Baptist Church.

In planning the Healing Springs Public School, a committee of six men was appointed. Only three—J. J. Ray, L. P. Boylston, and B. P. Boylston—attended the planning meeting. Ballots were cast in a tin can and Lute Boylston took the ballots to the Barnwell County Court House. Lute owned a sawmill and offered to give half the lumber for the two-story school building. Jeff Whittle gave the other half, plus the land. In the 1940s this school would be consolidated into the Blackville school system. Today, the building serves as a Mennonite school.

News trickled into Blackville about the many wonderful things happening elsewhere in the nation and around the world. People visiting or traveling through town in 1904 told about the great St. Louis fair. They described new foods and drinks such as ice cream cones, hamburgers, and iced tea. Others told of the Wright brothers' airplane flight at Kitty Hawk, North Carolina, in 1903. From newspapers they learned about the war between Japan and Russia. Having experienced the great Charleston earthquake, Healing Springs and Blackville citizens felt great sympathy for those living in San Francisco during the earthquake of 1906.

As in summers past, Healing Springs and Blackville residents spent long, hot days at picnics and retreats, some on the banks of the South Edisto River, near Boylston Landing and Holman's Bridge. They camped for a week at a time, enjoying fish fries and barbecues. They swam in the cool, black waters of the South Edisto River. In the evenings, after supper, they gathered around campfires, sat on logs and sang songs. Some of the songs they enjoyed were "Ida, Sweet as Apple Cider," "Sweet Adeline," "Wait Till the Sun Shines, Nellie," and "In the Shade of the Old Apple Tree."

More and more people were buying automobiles like the Model T Ford. Some of the first in the area to make this purchase were rural mail carriers and physicians. Although less than two percent of all farm families owned cars, there were about 200,000 cars on the road across the nation. As more automobiles came into use, there was more freedom of travel. Young adults, in particular, welcomed the opportunity to escape the watchful eyes of their parents.

In Blackville new businesses sprang up along Railroad Avenue. Mail order business began to boom. Sears Roebuck distributed over three million catalogs in 1907. As new editions arrived, the old Sears catalogs were useful in outhouses.

Still, there was not much money for most people to buy goods. The average pay for American workers in 1910 was less than $15 per week for fifty-four to sixty hours of work.

Over the years, the springs continued to flow. Water was there for all to drink. Generation after generation visited the springs and drank the healing waters. Throughout the centuries, the springs have been owned by six people. Nathaniel Walker originally purchased from the Indians. Walker sold the springs to Lester Woodward, who in turn sold the springs to Capt. P. W. Farrell, who sold to a Mr. Heflin. After Heflin was killed, the springs were returned to Captain Farrell who auctioned them off, selling to Jeff Whittle. The final owner, Lute (Lucian P.) Boylston, purchased the springs from Whittle about 1900.

Lute Boylston made attempts to commercialize the springs. At one point, a resort hotel was built—as was being done near other such artesian springs around the nation. But the hotel idea failed. In 1907, Lute and his brother Belton decided to open a bottling plant and sell soft drinks. This was the time that Coca-Cola, Dr. Pepper, and White Rock sparkling water were increasing in popularity. They built their bottling plant to the east side of the springs. From Germany they purchased thick blown glass bottles with rounded concave bottoms, like wine bottles, which could withstand the carbon dioxide gas pressure. The operation was completely manual, including labeling and capping. Some of the flavors sold included strawberry, pineapple, orange, chocolate, ginger ale, root beer, and sarsaparilla. Dealers paid 70 cents per case of twenty-four bottles and retailers sold each bottle for 5 cents. The Boylston brothers transported their drinks by wagon to local businesses and by train to Charleston and Columbia. Some Healing Springs water was sold and shipped in large demijohns. After about three years it became apparent to the brothers they could not compete with the large soft drink companies and closed up shop. That was the last time Healing Springs water was sold commercially.

Around the turn of the century, over two million blacks left the South for northern factories. At the time, eight out of every ten blacks in the United States still lived in the South. In an effort to improve opportunities for the country's black citizens the National Association for the Advancement of Colored People (NAACP) was founded in 1910.

Around the world, there were tragedies. In 1912, news reached America about the sinking of the *Titanic*, with 1,513 lives lost. There were rumors of wars around the globe—of course, these seemed so far away, across the ocean, they were of little concern.

The 1920s were good years by and large for those living in Blackville and Healing Springs. Compared to the rest of the United States, however, the South was still very poor. Considering where the South was at the end of the Civil War, one could see significant progress for most white people. Blacks would likely have made similar progress had it not been for "Jim Crow."

It is difficult for those living outside the South in the 1920s to understand how good, religious white people allowed segregation. To most Blackville and Healing Springs whites, segregation was accepted with complaisance. Older whites had known the blacks in the community since they were slaves and felt their situation was the result of being set free. As free men, they had to make their own way in life. Unfortunately blacks did not have the same opportunities as whites. Segregation took away the ability of many blacks to succeed personally or professionally—in the South as well as other parts of the nation.

Possibly, there remained an undercurrent of fear by many whites. Because of the large black population in the

South, there had for generations existed a fear of a revolt. "Jim Crow" laws were passed in an effort to dominate and control blacks and keep them in "their places." Today, it is easy to see the deficiencies of segregation—for our white ancestors living in the 1920s and 1930s it was not so easy to see. In those days, men in powerful positions sometimes remained so for years, and most people did not challenge the powers that be as readily as we do today. Many simply—blindly—followed the leaders. When whites heard of lynching, they chose to believe the blacks did something wrong and deserved it. It would take fifty years for the offenders to realize they had been wrong.

For the most part, blacks and whites living and working together around Blackville and Healing Springs had good relationships, especially farmers. Black sharecroppers were treated fairly by most farm owners—although there were isolated cases of wrongdoing. Young blacks leaving the farms for the North evidenced the main protest against segregation. Most whites who could afford it hired blacks to cook, clean house, and work in the yard. In rural areas, black and white children usually played together—that changed when they became teenagers and segregation caused them to go their separate ways. Most whites who were children in the 1920s and 1930s remember special black people who influenced their lives. Despite segregation, these bonds have lasted a lifetime. Possibly it is because of these good memories and childhood experiences some black Americans felt at home returning to the South in later life.

Significant changes took place in the nation as it

moved into the 1920s. The Prohibition Law passed on January 29, 1919, and in the years that followed people tried to figure out what to do about it. Those who drank whiskey were not about to stop. They determined to make their own if necessary. This was the beginning of the bootleg business, which grew and remained prosperous until Prohibition was repealed in 1933.

On August 26, 1920, women won the right to vote. It had been a long struggle—which included many family arguments around private dinner tables. This was the first step in a battle for equal rights for women, which continues today.

Another national milestone was reached in 1921 when for the first time urban population surpassed rural. Although the nation was only fifty-one percent urban, this was a significant change. As the population of cities increased so did economic problems. Rural areas experienced their own economic troubles with farm surpluses. More cotton was grown to increase farm income. This resulted in an excess that drove the market price down. Farmers were selling more cotton, but making the same money. In 1929, Congress passed the Agricultural Marketing Act, which established a Federal Farm Board to help farmers sell their surplus products.

The world continued to appear to shrink as had happened when the railroad first came to Blackville. Now, with the telegraph, telephone, radio, automobile, and airplane, news traveled rapidly to every corner of the United States. Rural Healing Springs and Blackville didn't seem so remote anymore. These were exciting times. America had become a wealthy nation and was prominent in the world. The first to sense this were the young adults. Their opportunities appeared unlimited. As they gathered on Saturday nights, they danced and sang the latest songs, such as, "Dark Eyes," "Take Me Out to the Ball Game," "It's a Long Way to Tipperary," "By the Light of the Silvery Moon," and "Put on Your Old Gray Bonnet."

Worldwide trouble finally affected Healing Springs and Blackville in 1914, when news reached the communities that war had begun in Europe. This would be a new type of war, with airplanes, poison gas, and tanks. The situation was grave. The media quoted British Secretary of State, Sir Edward Grey, as saying, "The lamps are going out all over Europe, and we shall not see them lit again in our lifetime." Soon there were German air raids over Paris.

Songs sung by young people took on a serious note and reflected their concerns of war: "Keep the Home Fires Burning," "There's a Long, Long Trail," and "Pack Up Your Troubles in Your Old Kit Bag." Over the next few years the war escalated, drawing the United States closer to the conflict. In 1917, after Germany declared unrestricted submarine warfare, the U. S. declared war on Germany. As the first American troops went to the front in France, popular songs indicated their plight: "Over There" and "You're in the Army Now."

Most young men around Healing Springs and Blackville volunteered or were drafted. Among those serving were the author's ancestor, George W. Boylston, Jr., and some of his cousins. There were 2.8 million inductees during this war. About 1.4 million served in France, where 116,516 were killed and 204,002 wounded. President Woodrow Wilson proclaimed the American "doughboys" would "make the world safe for democracy."

Meetings and rallies were held in Blackville to promote support for the war. Liberty bonds were sold and war posters displayed in most businesses. One prominent piece of promotion was Uncle Sam's "I Want You" draft poster. Everyone was urged to conserve food, and "meatless days" were practiced.

Healing Springs and Blackville citizens were much more fortunate during World War I than they had been during the Civil War. The main evidence of war was the uniform of young men visiting home. After the war ended in November 1918, evidence of the war remained, as some soldiers returning home were disabled from wounds or gas exposure.

The European war had convinced most Americans, including those living in Healing Springs and Blackville, that the United States should stay out of foreign conflicts. Not only had over 116,000 young men been killed, but the national debt rose from a pre-war $1 billion to $26.5 billion. President Wilson toured the country in an unsuccessful attempt to get citizen support for joining the League of Nations. While on this tour, the president suffered a stroke.

The aftermath of World War I led to the country's greatest economic depression in the early 1930s and to world unrest that lead to the rise of Communism, Fascism, and Nazism.

Possibly, the thing that hit communities around Healing Springs hardest was not the war and its aftermath but
the flu. One of the world's greatest influenza epidemics
hit 1918-19. About 20 million Americans died in this epidemic. Since the viral infection was spread by contact with
others, most rural residents were spared the worst. People
had learned during the Civil War to avoid large crowds
and keep their distance during such epidemics. There were
a few deaths in Barnwell County, but nothing to compare
to large cities.

In an effort for America to isolate itself more from
the rest of the world, Congress raised tariff duties in 1922
to the highest level seen to that time. This shut out most
foreign goods entering the United States. This high tariff
hit Healing Springs and Blackville farmers harder than
World War I and the flu epidemic. Farmers had increased
their production of cash crops and now had no place to
sell them. Farm income fell from $15 billion to $5.5 billion. Pressure was put on Congress to improve the
farmer's plight, but President Calvin Coolidge vetoed
plans to raise farm prices twice. The farmers were left to
solve their own problems. Most did as they had done in
the past—they cut back to producing just what they needed
to survive, waiting for better times.

While the farmers were hurting, the rest of the nation
enjoyed the "roaring twenties"—it was "Happy Days are
Here Again" and "Let the Good Times Roll." For the first
time, there were nationwide youth uprisings. Bold young
people shocked their elders by revolting against pre-war
standards. Flappers were everywhere, with bobbed hair,

"cloche" hats, rolled silk stockings, shorter skirts, long sweaters, necklaces, and open galoshes. Many smoked cigarettes. Model T Fords were everywhere and a few Stutz Bearcats. It was a time of *ballyhoo* and *whoopee*. Everything "normal" was under assault. Young people fled rural areas for the large cities.

The slow pace of small-town America was under attack. Automobiles, radios, magazines, and motion pictures provided more contact with the outside world and a breakaway from family ties. The rural way of life was being eroded. However, change came at a slower pace in rural areas. Automobiles gave freedom of movement. The radio brought all types of music, more humor, and better speech into the home. The young were quick to absorb this new information. Songs of the time included "I'll See You in My Dreams," "It Had to be You," "Yes Sir! That's My Baby," "Sweet Georgia Brown," "Always," and "Me and My Shadow."

News arrived over the radio and in newspapers about the threat of Communism in America. To most southerners, this was a big city problem and didn't worry them too much. The new Ku Klux Klan, however, was a threat. Many local citizens in Blackville and neighboring towns joined the Klan and attended meetings. Initially, the mission of the group seemed to be trying to stop what the members perceived as outside corruption. The Klan was anti everything—anti-foreign, anti-Catholic, anti-Semitic, anti-Negro, anti-urban. This movement was widespread, with an estimated five million members. After a few years, most members began to realize it was the wrong approach to solving the nation's problems. There were a number of scandals involving the Klan that led to its downfall.

Motion pictures were also bringing new ideas to small town America. Women dreamed of Rudolph Valentino carrying them off across the desert. For the young, there were Tom Mix westerns. During these early days of film, there were no theaters, so traveling movie companies set up in towns, showing movies on screens in rented buildings or, if the weather was good, in open areas.

It was a time of flagpole sitting, crossword puzzles, card games such as contract bridge, and the "Charleston," a dance that originated in the "Holy City." There was also sports, and some of the greats were looked on as idols: Babe Ruth, Lou Gehrig, Bobby Jones, Red Grange, and Jack Dempsey.

At the same time styles and attitudes were lossening, there was a religious revival. Outstanding preachers like Billy Sunday and Aimee Semple McPherson offered strong messages of God's Word. Encouraged by this renewed interest in religion, the Healing Springs and Blackville churches brought in visiting preachers and held revivals, open to everyone.

In May 1927 Americans shouted with joy when they learned of Charles A. Lindbergh's solo flight across the Atlantic Ocean to Paris in a single-engine monoplane. Lindbergh was truly an American hero. Big progress was made in fighting diseases when penicillin was discovered in 1928. The significance of this discovery would not be realized until the second world war. The Majestic radio, a significant improvement over existing models was produced that same year. Unknown to most people, the first television broadcast was made in 1928. It would take another thirty years before the full impact of this medium would be felt.

The crash of Wall Street in 1929 marked an indication of things to come. At that time, seventy-one percent of the nation's families had annual average incomes below $2,500. The average weekly wage was $28. Half of all farm families produced less than $1,000 worth of food, cotton, or tobacco each year.

As the 1930s began, young people still gathered at their favorite spots, enjoying each other's company and singing the latest songs—"I'll Get By," "Carolina Moon," "Star Dust," and "Honeysuckle Rose." Ordinary people didn't suspect what lay ahead.

The soil along the South Edisto River and the other streams in the area was fertile, flat, free of rock or hard pan, and perfect for agriculture. Good rainfall followed the river. Good agriculture and good railroad transportation made Blackville a natural farmers' market. From the early 1800s to the late 1920s cotton remained the main money crop. In 1926, 29,244 bales of cotton were ginned in Barnwell County. In 1925, there were 1,340 railcar loads of watermelons, 28 cars of cantaloupes, and 400 cars of cucumbers shipped from the county, most from Blackville. About 200 railcars loaded with asparagus shipped from the Blackville-Williston area in 1926. Other produce shipped included beans, squash, tomatoes, potatoes, cabbage, lettuce, and peas. During the late 1920s and into the 1930s, Blackville was a thriving agricultural market-place. The entire street on the north side of the railroad was an open-air market. Wagons, trucks, and trailers parked side by side as hundreds of people engaged in selling and buying produce. Farmers from a fifteen-mile area surrounding Blackville brought their products to the Blackville market. The author hauled cantaloupes from Springfield to the Blackville market in 1946 and personally saw the significance of the market.

Dan Ross of Blackville described to the author how he and his uncle, Percy Beasley, worked at the market during summers loading watermelons into railroad boxcars. His uncle was an expert watermelon packer. Dan and his friends would toss the watermelons up to his uncle for proper packing. That's how Dan built up his arm strength for playing football.

Percy Beasley also drove a homemade school bus in the early 1930s. The families of school children paid $4 a month for each child transported to and from school. Dan said his father borrowed the old school bus and drove his family to Holman's Bridge where they camped out after the fields were cleared in the summer. As the years went by, Holman's Bridge grew in popularity as a recreational area. The bridge had closed in the early 1900s and the new Highway 3 bridges, replacing Duncan's Bridge, opened between Blackville and Springfield.

THE GREAT DEPRESSION

Since the small farmers around Healing Springs and Blackville had lived through so many difficult times—establishing homes in the wilderness, Indian attacks, Tory brutality, Sherman's bummers, droughts, the boll weevil—they probably were better prepared than most to handle the great depression of the 1930s. They were survivors and knew how to live on very little.

Economic crisis resulted when a significant increase in industrial production in the 1920s failed to bring an equal rise in wages. While business owners were reaping huge profits, the average citizen could not afford to buy the products being made. Encouraged by advertisements, they bought goods on the new installment plan. For a while everything looked great and the good times kept rolling. Finally, as monthly installment payments could not be met, people stopped purchasing. The factories kept producing, however, glutting the market. Then came a slowdown in production and worker layoffs. Layoffs resulted in less money to pay bills and make purchases. Before long, the country was in the midst of a depression.

The Wall Street crash of 1929 was followed by another in 1930. Four million U. S. workers were unemployed. Thirteen hundred banks closed. And all this happened during one of the worst droughts in Healing Springs history. Farmers were hard hit. In 1930, about twenty-five percent of all Americans still lived on farms with an annual average income of $400. Forty percent of the farms were still worked by tenant farmers who made just enough income to survive. Many of the farmers near Blackville and Healing Springs had borrowed heavily and mortgaged their farms to buy new and more efficient farm machinery. Their debts had increased by two-thirds since 1910.

Farmers gathered around their Majestic radios after supper and listened to national and world events from announcer Lowell Thomas. The news Thomas reported about the stock market crash didn't concern most listeners since very few, if any, owned stock. Also, the country had been through crashes in 1873, 1893, and 1907 and recovered. Reports of the drought and bank closings did concern them however. What scared them most were reports of farmers losing their farms because of defaulting on taxes.

Healing Springs and Blackville farmers were a close-knit group. They stuck together during tough times. As farm mortgage foreclosures were announced, they all gathered at the sales, brandishing pitchforks, axes, and shotguns to threaten the sheriff and save the farms. Backed by his neighbors, who prevented others from bidding, the desperate farmer redeemed his forfeited farm for a few dollars.

Along with the bad news about the economy, in 1931, *The State* newspaper reported that Japan had invaded Manchuria. Everyone had had enough war and prayed the U. S. would not become involved again. Americans were still feeling the repercussions from World War

I. Because of the depression, World War I veterans began asking that the bonus they had been promised be paid to them early. In July 1932 thousands of vets marched on Washington and camped out at the White House demanding their money. The U. S. Army drove the marchers out of the capital. In November of that same year Franklin D. Roosevelt was elected president. At that time there were 13 million unemployed workers in the country.

In 1933 Adolph Hitler assumed office as chancellor of Germany. Most people had never heard of him and knew little about him. All that would change over the next five years.

Roosevelt began his attack on the depression by declaring a bank holiday. Congress passed the Reformation Relief Act, which established the Civilian Conservation Corps (CCC). Over 250,000 young men joined up, each receiving $30 per month. By the beginning of World War II, two million men had served in the CCC. The CCC turned out to be a good training program for the army.

A flood of "New Deal" acts to increase employment and end the depression were passed by Congress between 1933 and 1935. These included the National Industrial Recovery Act (NIRA), which established the Public Works Administration (PWA) and the National Recovery Administration (NRA). In 1935 the Supreme Court would declare the NRA unconstitutional.

Congress did not leave the farmers out. In 1934 they passed the Farm Mortgage Refinancing Act and the Cotton Control Act. The Refinancing Act provided easy credit to farmers. The Cotton Control Act set mandatory controls on cotton production. Later that same year, the Farm Mortgage Foreclosure Act was passed. This helped farmers recover their farms.

In 1935, Congress passed a number of significant acts to help farmers and other laborers. That April, the Soil Conservation Service was established to protect farmland. Then in May, Congress passed the Works Progress Administration (WPA). This program was probably the best known of all developed to help people during the depression. Some made fun of the WPA, saying it stood for "We Poke Along." The majority of people, however, felt the program produced good results. Millions were put to work at reasonable wages building roads, bridges, and thousands of public structures such as schools, gymnasiums, post offices, parks, and airfields. The program also provided employment for artists, musicians, actors, writers, and scholars. The program continued until 1943, employing 8.5 million workers. Considering workers' need to retire as they aged, Roosevelt signed the Social Security Act in August 1935.

While America struggled through the depression, events of note were happening in other parts of the world. Of great concern was the Spanish Civil War. The media reported the bombing of Spanish cities by German bombers and the slaughter of civilians, including women and children. A number of Americans volunteered to go to Spain and assist in the war effort.

King Edward VIII of Great Britain surprised the world by abdicating his throne to marry American divorcee Wallis Warfield Simpson. In the summer of 1936 black American Jesse Owens became the pride of his country with his triumphs in Track and Field at the Olympic games in Berlin.

Urban America experienced more change during the depression than rural America. Most large cities had long bread lines and many homeless people on the streets. Beggars were everywhere and hobos traveled in freight cars on every train. Healing Springs and Blackville remained fundamentally sound. They could grow their own food and store it. They knew how to use local waterways to their advantage. Times were tough, but they had experienced tough times before and knew their hard work and strong faith would see them through. They focused on improving education as a way to better life for themselves and for their children.

The period's writers—Willa Cather, William Faulkner, F. Scott Fitzgerald, Ernest Hemingway, Sinclair Lewis, and Carl Sandburg—wrote about the conditions in America. One Southern writer from North Carolina was a master at describing life in the South in the 1920s and 1930s: Thomas Wolfe of Asheville. In *Look Homeward, Angel* he wrote about small towns like Blackville: "There is a smell of burning in small towns in the afternoon, and men with buckles on their arms are raking leaves in yards as boys come by with straps slung back across their shoulders. The oak leaves, big and brown, are bedded deep in yard and gutter: they make deep wading to the knees for children in the streets. The fire will snap and crackle like a whip, sharp acrid smoke will sting the eyes, in mown fields the little vipers of the flame eat past the black coarse edges of burned stubble like a line of locust. Fire drives a thorn of memory in the heart."

Bill Odom described to the author some of his experiences around Healing Springs in the 1930s. He and his friends swam in the Healing Springs Baptist Church baptismal pool. Many were later baptized in the same pool, which was fed by cold spring water. Some people said the cold spring water would "freeze your sins away." At home Frank Odom, Bill's father, and his brothers sang together and played their guitars and banjos. Often these sing-alongs included peanut boilings and watermelon cuttings.

At Christmas time, Healing Springs boys shot firecrackers. Like most young boys, they were full of mischief and sometimes got into trouble. One night cherry bombs were tossed on porches of some area homes, including Mrs. Leila Gardner's. Leila was the wife of Bennett Gardner and a patriarch of the community. On that particular night, when the cherry bombs exploded, Miss Leila was quick to respond. She ran to the front door and, as she opened it, spotted Bill's cousin, R. B. Morris. "It's the Odom boys!" she shouted. She was right—a few Odom boys were in the bunch. This was one of many pranks the "Healing Springs" boys played. Sometimes they would crawl under houses, stick straws up through the cracks in the floor, and move them around. One person they frightened was Bill Odom's aunt, Jumelle Boylston.

When the local boys were not playing pranks on people, they visited Heckle's Store. Mr. Heckle always wore a suit, tie, watch chain, and hat. He was gruff, but kind to the boys buying penny candy and drinks. Mr. Heckle was a former minister and member of the South Carolina House of Representatives. He was well educated and informed. Local folks enjoyed talking with him and listening to his opinions.

Bill Odom also remembered some of his failed ventures during the 1920s and 1930s. One included a resort hotel built about a half mile from Healing Springs, on the road to Blackville. Another was a recreation area with a large swimming pool situated about two miles north of the springs, developed with help from the WPA.

Despite the depression, small-town life continued as normal as possible. Young people still played baseball and swam in the creeks, ponds, and South Edisto River. They gathered and sang and danced to the latest tunes. This was the Big Band era, which gave us lively music. Thanks to radio and phonographs, everyone could enjoy the music. "Mood Indigo," "Brother Can You Spare a Dime," "We're in the Money," "Life is just a Bowl of Cherries," and "Where the Blue of the Night Meets the Gold of the Day," sung by Bing Crosby, were just a few of the popular songs. As young people listened to swing music, the older folks were listening to the radio broadcast of *Lum and Abner*. The newspapers now carried comic strips, which included "Mickey Mouse" by Walt Disney.

The depression worsened and another radio news broadcaster's voice became familiar. Walter Winchell began each report with, "Good evening, Mr. and Mrs. America and all the ships at sea." Every evening, after supper, farm families gathered around the radio for Winchell's report. Fathers generally sat next to the small table radio where he had control of the dials. All the kids knew to keep quiet and listen to everything that was said. After Winchell signed off, families often discussed what was said.

President Roosevelt began his "Fireside Chats" in 1938. These broadcasts kept Americans informed about the depression and what was being done. Roosevelt told everyone "the only thing we have to fear, is fear itself." It was about this time that radio programs, like *Buck Rogers*, began to broadcast in the afternoon after school for youngsters.

The prices of farm products fell to forty percent of their 1929 level. Cotton was selling for five cents per pound. Farmers who were not in debt decided to store their cotton in barns and warehouses until the prices rose again. Small farmers, of course, could not afford to do this.

Although most Americans were more concerned about local and national affairs, they listened to the disturbing news from overseas. In 1933, Adolf Hitler began his dictatorship of Germany and Japan withdrew from the League of Nations.

Americans tried to forget their problems by reading, listening to the radio, and singing songs such as, "How Deep is the Ocean," "Basin Street Blues," and "Only a Paper Moon." A favorite pastime was going to the picture show to see the moving pictures, like *Stand Up and Cheer*, Shirley Temple's first full-length film at age six. Those who couldn't afford the five cents for the movie listened to *Lux Radio Theater*.

In the mid 1930s, the Civilian Conservation Corps (CCC) built a number of South Carolina state parks, including Aiken and Barnwell. New school buildings and gyms were built, some of which are still in use today. Many families would not have had enough to eat had it not been for the wages made from employment in the government programs. School lunches began to be served during this period.

Walter Winchell reported in 1934 that Bonnie and Clyde had been killed in Louisiana and John Dillinger killed in Chicago. New advertisements announced Royal Crown Cola. On August 15, 1935, America's beloved Will Rogers and his friend, pilot Wiley Post, were killed in a plane crash in Alaska.

One of the most important events of this decade was passage of the Rural Electrification Act (REA) in 1935. At that time only ten percent of the country's thirty million rural residents had electrical service. With electricity, the overall standard of living for farm families greatly improved over the next ten years.

However, most farmers in the 1930s still used kerosene lamps and lanterns. Houses were still heated by fireplaces or iron stoves. Water was pumped manually with hand pumps or hauled in buckets from open wells. A few farms had installed windmills to pump water into elevated wooden tanks. Baths were taken in round tin tubs with water warmed on iron stoves. Behind every house was a woodpile or wood shed and nearby an outhouse with the old reliable Sears Roebuck catalog. Houses were usually unpainted clapboard structures with wood shingle or tin roofs. Many houses had no screens at windows or doors. Safes (cabinets with screen doors) were used in kitchens to keep flies and other insects off the food. The walls and floors were thin, with no insulation, making the houses hot in summer and cold in winter. It was not uncommon for people to heat bricks by stoves and wrap them in blankets for children to take to bed to keep them warm. This was done because there was no heat in the bedrooms. During the summer, children slept with their beds pushed to open windows. They fell asleep listening to the hoot of owls. Contrary to popular belief, the roosters crowed in the middle of the night as well as at daybreak.

During the 1930s Christmas was extra special. Maybe it was because of the depression, but people seemed more involved in holiday festivities. Most of the year, there was little to celebrate and much hard work just to make ends meet. However, at Christmas the whole atmosphere seemed to change. There were more smiles on people's faces and folks were friendlier. Children could sense the change and got caught up in the Christmas spirit.

A few days before Christmas, fathers and grandfathers hiked with the children into nearby woods to cut a Christmas tree, usually a cedar. Some people used small pines or holly trees covered with red berries. Decorating the tree was a family affair. Children made paper chains from strips of colored paper "glued" together with homemade flour paste. Popcorn was strung into long ropes with needle and thread. Aluminum icicles were carefully removed from a shoebox where they had been saved from last year's tree. Cotton balls were placed on the tree's limbs. Each child would make a special paper Christmas ornament and color it with crayons. A white paper star was placed on top of the tree. Finally, a cotton sheet was placed under the tree to simulate snow. Once the tree was complete, everyone stood back and admired it, always saying it was the most beautiful Christmas tree ever.

Healing Springs Baptist Church and the First Baptist Church of Blackville always had special holiday programs, usually involving the children. The choirs practiced for weeks perfecting their Christmas songs. At candlelight services, each person held a small candle as everyone sang carols. To the children this was quite impressive. They would remember the candles and songs for the rest of their lives.

Each person received one small Christmas gift. Often, these were homemade items—toys for the children and clothes for the adults. All were thankful for what they received, knowing they were more fortunate than many. It was not the gifts but the Christmas spirit that really made everyone happy. Today's old-timers, who were children in the 1930s, look back on those days as one of the happiest periods of their lives.

Despite the hard work in keeping the farms going, there was time for fun, especially during the long summer months. Each town had a baseball team and each high school a football team. Young boys joined the Boy Scouts of America. During the late 1930s a group of fifteen Blackville Boy Scouts—including D. I. Ross, Jack Boylston, and W. S. (Buck) Guess, ages eleven to fifteen, built a log scout hut. Other scouts involved in the project were

Buddy Davis, Charles Carroll, and Jack O'Gorman. Crum Boylston, a local hardware store owner, donated tin for the roof and concrete for the floor. When the scouts were not working on their log hut, they were camping on the banks of the South Edisto River.

Businesses in Blackville in the mid to late 1930s included Simon Brown's Sons Inc. (general merchandise), Poliakoff's, Wiengow's, Blatt's, Kaplan's, O'Gorman's, Morrison's, and Turner's. Nathan Blatt, a Jewish immigrant from Russia, walked from Charleston to Blackville and opened a dry goods store (Blatt's). Once his business became successful, he brought his wife and son Jake over from Russia. They built a home on Clark Street where Solomon Blatt was born. Sol Blatt would later become one of South Carolina's leading politicians. H. L. Buist operated a "picture show" on Main Street next to the old post office. J. L. Buist, the Hoffmans, Dora Hutto, Willie McCormack, Sam G. Lowe, Sam Buist, and Ben Creech operated grocery stores. McDonalds Superette opened after Buist grocery store closed. Sem and C. A. Epps owned pharmacies. Clyde and Lizzie Boylston ran a hardware store. Ben Boylston's and Simon Brown's sons operated livery stables. There was also Boylston's furniture store.

The community around the Healing Springs Baptist Church stopped growing after the town of Blackville developed around the railroad stop. Today, there are about the same number of homes around the springs as there were seventy years ago. Some of the people living there during the depression included Lute Boylston, Murry and Ellen Odom, Mozelle and Shannon Williams, Rev. Ben

Gardner, Gladys Breeden, Minnie Odom, Frank Odom, and Jumelle Odom Boylston. On the corner of the Healing Springs Road and the Springfield-Blackville Road was Heckle's Store. As in the past, the church remains the focal point of community life. During the day there is a steady flow of vehicles of all descriptions traveling to and from the springs. Visitors are also of all descriptions: men, women, children, young, old, black, white, rich, poor, healthy, ill. They come from far and near for the healing water. They drink generously of the cool water, then fill their tin buckets, glass jugs, plastic jugs, wooden barrels, and metal containers. At night, when all are gone, the clear, cool, healing waters continue flowing. Then the deer, raccoons, foxes, squirrels, opposums, and other woodland creatures partake of the water. The cycle of life at Healing Springs continues as it has for thousands of years.

As testimony to Blackville's progress in the 1930s, there were four physicians—Hammond, Gyles, Briggs, and Kneece—and three dentists—Molony, Strone, and Buist.

Race relations had not improved by the 1930s. If anything, they had grown worse with the depression, which hit most black Carolinians harder than most whites. Whites continued to ensure that blacks were kept in "their place." Lynchings continued with little, if any, objection from anyone. South Carolina newspapers usually condoned lynching and offered little sympathy for black victims. Protests by blacks were generally ignored.

Farmers began to diversify by planting peanuts, soybeans, watermelons, cantaloupes, cucumbers, and asparagus. The town of Williston, South Carolina, became an asparagus-growing center while Blackville was a cucumber center. Efforts were made to put hard surfaces on dirt farm-to-market roads. The first Monday of each month was "sales day," when farmers carried produce and livestock to town to sell. In this way they made enough money to keep from borrowing from the bank.

Saturday was the best day of the week. Those with money went to town to make purchases and have fun. Most small farmers still did not own automobiles. They rode to town in mule-drawn buggies and wagons, which they tied behind stores. Those driving automobiles parked along the street. Shoppers crowded the sidewalks. Small children earned about 25 cents per week doing special chores around home and they spent it on Saturday. An ice cream cone cost 5 cents; a bag of boiled peanuts, 5 cents; and a seat at the movies, 15 cents. On Saturday afternoons there were always cowboy movies. In those days everyone tried to get as close to the screen as they could. Once the lights were turned off there was usually a cartoon, then a continuing serial like *The Lone Ranger* or *Flash Gordon*, and then the movie. The most popular cowboy stars—before the singing cowboys like Gene Autry and Roy Rogers—were The Three Musketeers, Hopalong Cassidy, and Bob Steele. Later, Tarzan movies and comedies were shown.

While youngsters went to the movies, adults gathered on the main street and discussed the weather and farm problems. Many of the men routinely visited the local barbershop on Saturday mornings where they could get a haircut for 25 cents, a shave for 25 cents, and a shoeshine for 5 cents. While waiting their turns, they talked to friends and played checkers or pool.

Wives usually shopped or sat in autos on the main street while their husbands talked with friends and the children went to the movie. Some women belonged to bridge clubs and met each Saturday afternoon at someone's house for refreshments and bridge. In general, living was easy and slow. They would have liked to have more, but decided to be content with what they had.

In 1936, there was significant news from overseas. King George V died at age seventy and was succeeded by his forty-one-year-old son Edward VIII, who abdicated the throne before year's end. Edward's brother George VI succeeded him. During that year Italy invaded Ethiopia, and Spain erupted in civil war. Not only was there fighting in Africa and Europe, but in Asia the Japanese invaded China. Little did Americans know, as they listened to Walter Winchell's radio news, that this fighting was only the beginning. While everyone was still mourning the death of Will Rogers, there was news of Amelia Earhart's disappearance while flying across the Pacific Ocean.

During this time *Mutiny on the Bounty, The Charge of the Light Brigade,* and *Trail of the Lonesome Pine* showed in the Blackville movie theater. And "I'm in the Mood for Love," "Moon Over Miami," "Red Sails in the Sunset," and "Good Night Irene" were popular songs on the radio. America's Big Bands—Benny Goodman, Glenn Miller, and Tommy and Jimmy Dorsey—continued to play and thrill listeners.

The radio broadcast of the Joe Lewis and Max Schmeling boxing match in 1938 got everyone's attention. Schmeling defeated Lewis in their first fight and now Lewis was ready for the return match, which he won.

For the younger children, there were the new Superman comic books. Soon many more comic books followed. Most boys kept them in a cardboard box to swap with friends. In 1938, Walt Disney released the first full-length animated cartoon feature film, *Snow White and the Seven Dwarfs*. Young people living around Healing Springs and Blackville were also good at creating their own entertainment. Young boys played cowboys and Indians and swung on ropes like Tarzan. They made their own bows and arrows and played Robin Hood.

Music was changing fast. Just prior to World War II, "One O'clock Jump," "The Flat Foot Floogie," and "A-Tisket, A-Tasket." As soon as America became involved in the war in Europe, the type of songs young people sang changed again.

THE SOUTH FORK OF THE EDISTO
By Jimmie Page Gunter

In memory I often go,
To a place I used to know,
Where quiet waters ebb and flow,
The South Fork of the Edisto.

We'd dig some worms and string our poles,
Then make our way to deep, dark holes,
Where bream and red horse breached the
flow,
The South Fork of the Edisto.

Friends came by for me to play, to be told
"Not here today!"
"Gone where quiet waters flow,
The South Fork of the Edisto."

Main Street often held forth signs,
Of gentle people, quieter times,
"Closed today, I had to go,"
"See you at the Edisto!"

If I could have one wish today,
I'd take my sweetheart's hand
And say,
"Let's pack a lunch, I need to go,"
"Fishing on the Edisto."

The decade of the thirties ended as it began, with worldwide disaster. 1939 marked the beginning of World War II in Europe. Radio news reports described the tragedy of Germany's invasion of Poland on September 1, 1939. Football practice at Blackville High School had just started and the young men were all on the practice field as the war news arrived. After practice, they gathered around the coach, asking questions about what had happened. Most of the young men had heard of Germany and Hitler, but were not sure where Poland was located. During the next five years most of them would learn much more about world geography—much of it firsthand in the Pacific and Europe. Everyone realized just how bad things were when, on September 3, Britain and France declared war on Germany. Not long after, the Russians invaded Poland and Finland.

A new voice traveled the airwaves from overseas. Edward R. Murrow began his *This is London* broadcast, bringing the war in Europe right to the sitting rooms of American families. For the first time people could hear the sounds of war as events happened. After the Murrow news reports, people listened to *The Chase and Sanborn Radio Hour* with Edgar Bergen and Charlie McCarthy and *The Dinah Shore Show*. The top movie of the year was *Gone With the Wind*, reminding everyone of another time and another war.

Soft drink companies were trying to outdo each other during this period. The greatest battle was between Pepsi-Cola and Coca-Cola. Pepsi came out with a snappy tune that got everyone's attention. "Pepsi-Cola hits the spot.

Twelve full ounces, that's a lot. Twice as much for a nickel, too. Pepsi-Cola is the drink for you."

Young Frank Sinatra was just beginning to get his start with the Harry James band in 1939 and young women were all in love with him. Hit songs reflected the war and mood of the country: "There'll Always Be an England" and "I'll Never Smile Again." Other popular numbers included "And the Angels Sing," "Moonlight Serenade," "In the Mood," "South of the Border," "Three Little Fishes," and "God Bless America."

Irvin Berlin wrote "God Bless America" in the fall of 1938. It was a revision of an earlier version. Singer Kate Smith introduced the song on Armistice Day 1938 and it was an immediate hit.

Although it is generally agreed that things were advanced by 1939, fewer than sixty percent of all Americans owned automobiles. This number was much lower in Barnwell County with only a few farmers owning cars. The income of Americans was still so low that only three percent had to pay any income tax.

Living through the depression of the 1930s made everyone appreciate what they had. All people had to do was look around, and they would see others who were worse off.

THE FORTIES

Despite great national advances and the high standard of living in most large cities, rural South Carolina was about twenty-five years behind. One could walk or ride down the streets of Blackville and see large, beautiful homes painted white with long porches across the front and well-kept yards.

Once you left town and headed for the country, the picture changed. While the main roads were paved in the 1930s, most side and connecting roads remained unpaved. The highway department used motorized road scrapers occasionally to smooth out potholes on connecting roads. But side roads were much like they were in the early 1800s—two-rut dirt paths. Some of these roads, which usually led to farm homes and fields, had sand about a foot deep.

Farmhouses were generally unpainted. Out back by the unpainted barn were lots for mules, cows, and pigs. Southern barns and lots were small compared to those on northern and western farms. Cribs, boxes, and bins were placed in the barns for storing oats, corn, and cottonseed meal. Some barns were full of hay and fodder. During rainy weather, the lots became a sea of mud and manure. Not far behind the house was the outhouse, which had been in use for many, many years.

Sharecropper houses were often tiny cabins, with leaning chimneys. The poorer ones had long wooden poles set at an angle against the chimney to brace it. Inside walls of some houses were covered with newspapers to keep out the cold wind in winter. There was a certain smell to the poorer sharecropper houses that came from burning trash behind the house mingled with the odor of grease from frying fatback. Many of the sharecropper houses had no wells so they had to haul water in buckets from a nearby farmer's house or a spring. As one traveled the county roads of South Carolina in the late 1940s, it was commonplace to see tumbled down tenant houses.

Despite the migration of young black Carolinians to the North, about seventy percent of all blacks in the United States still lived in the South. In the forties, most of these were older sharecroppers. There remained about 6 million farms in the United States, 2.2 million of which were less than fifty acres apiece.

As a little more spending money became available for entertainment, more people were able to spend fifteen cents to see the movies of the day: *Grapes of Wrath* and *Waterloo Bridge*. On Saturday nights, young adults gathered as usual at their favorite places to listen and dance to "The Last Time I Saw Paris," "Bless 'em All," "Beat Me Daddy, Eight to the Bar," "Back in the Saddle Again," and "You Are My Sunshine."

Children on farms made their own entertainment. They went barefoot from the end of the school year until school started again in the fall. As the summer progressed, feet became tough, but sandspurs, ringworm, and hookworm caused some problems. Boys wore only short pants. Girls wore dresses made from cotton flour sacks, generally a floral print. Most young people living on farms remember being chased by cows, goats, ducks, geese, roosters, and hogs. They learned to keep alert when animals were around. There was always the concern about "mad dogs," as rabies treatment was not given then.

Malaria, whooping cough, polio, tetanus, typhoid fever, and chicken pox posed health problems. Mustard plasters were applied to the chests of children as people had done seventy-five years before. Most people around Healing Springs and Blackville who were children in the 1930s and 1940s remember taking quinine to ward off malaria. As a result of this treatment all food tasted like quinine during the summer.

The economy of Healing Springs and Blackville was still troubled, but folks believed President Roosevelt would see them through. Roosevelt won a second term and continued his "Fireside Chats." More tragic news arrived from overseas: the Germans had rushed through France, Belgium, the Netherlands, Denmark, and Norway.

When America's first peacetime military draft began on October 29, 1940, local citizens realized the wars in Europe and Asia were going to involve the United States. Soon, many young men would be leaving home as their fathers had done during World War I and their grandfathers and great-grandfathers had done during the Civil War. Each generation seemed to have its own war. As young men joined the army and navy, unemployment rolls decreased. However, there were still about 8 million Americans unemployed.

In Europe the war was progressing for the worst. The

battle of the Atlantic with the German U-boats was underway. In Britain, Winston Churchill succeeded Neville Chamberlain as Prime Minister. As thousands of British and French troops retreated to Dunkirk, Churchill proclaimed, "We shall fight on the beaches, we shall fight on the landing grounds, we shall fight in the fields and in the streets. . . . we shall never surrender!" Soon the German Luftwaffe began air attacks on the British Isles, starting the battle of Britain. When the British fighters drove them back, Churchill said, "Never in the field of human conflict was so much owed by so many to so few."

As 1941 began, most people felt things were better than they had been for many years. More people had jobs and more money was available. Everyone prayed the conflict in Europe would soon end. However, news of Germany attacking Russia meant the war was continuing to spread. All hope of peace came to an end on December 7, 1941, when the Japanese attacked the American fleet at Pearl Harbor in the Hawaiian Islands. "December 7 is a day that will live in infamy," President Roosevelt stated, addressing Congress the next day. This attack convinced Americans it was necessary to go to war. This would be a people's war, fought by citizen soldiers, paid for by Congress, and directed by elected citizen officials.

One of the first things people wanted to know was "Where is Pearl Harbor?" Many thought it was on the west coast of the United States. There were some quick geography lessons. President Roosevelt advised everyone to consult a world atlas and learn where the fighting was taking place. Now, people were speaking names and talking about places they had never heard about before Pearl Harbor.

As war industries began to increase production, the depression ended. Most people had jobs. When a shortage of male workers developed, more women entered the workforce. This would aid in the long, hard struggle of women for equal rights. Soon, about one-third of the United States economy was war-related. Increased employment brought increased prosperity and an improved standard of living, even in South Carolina.

During this period thousands of young men from Barnwell County entered service. Almost every home had a small banner with a blue star in the center hanging in a window, indicating a husband or son in service. It was a time of goodbyes, not only for soldiers, but also for many family members leaving home and the farm for industrial factories and other war-related jobs. Over 12 million men and women entered the armed services while about 15 million civilians took defense jobs.

Since the immigration of white Europeans in the 1500s, America had seen its share of conflict: the French and Indian War, the Regulator Revolt, the Revolution, the War of 1812, the Mexican War, the Civil War, the Spanish-American War, World War I, and now World War II. As with World War I, each evening farm families gathered around their radios, listening to news broadcasts. They heard terrifying reports of the Japanese sweeping across Southeast Asia and the South Pacific and the Germans driving the Russians back toward Moscow.

Popular songs reflected the war mood: "There'll Be

Blue Birds Over the White Cliffs of Dover," "Boogie Woogie Bugle Boy," and "Lili Marlene." Other songs were "Blues in the Night," "Elmer's Tune," and "Racing with the Moon." Some movies, like *Sergeant York*, had a war theme. Other films were American epics: *Citizen Kane* and *How Green was my Valley*.

By 1942, some good news began to arrive in Healing Springs and Blackville. For the first time the Allied armies were taking the offensive. Britain stopped the German advance in North Africa at El Alamein. A few months later, on November 7 and 8, Allied forces landed in North Africa. As this was happening, the Russians counterattacked at Stalingrad. Over the following months the Allies would push the Germans out of North Africa.

There was also some good news from the Pacific. Maj. James (Jimmy) Doolittle led an air raid on Tokyo with sixteen B-25 bombers, flown off an aircraft carrier. Barnwell County felt it had made a contribution to this raid since Doolittle and his men, who were stationed at Columbia, trained at the Barnwell Army Air Base.

America began a nationwide rationing with food stamps for sugar and stickers for gasoline. An "A" gas sticker allowed four gallons of gas per week. Everyone was encouraged to plant "victory gardens." Unemployment was continuing to drop—only 3.6 million remained unemployed in 1942.

Local citizens served as spotters for airplanes, calling in to designated phone numbers reports of airplanes flying overhead. Reports would begin with "Army flash 9105." People from Blackville and Healing Springs visiting

Charleston during this time saw firsthand the acts of war. German U-boats were sinking ships all along the east coast. At night all windows in houses and buildings along the coast were covered and outside lights turned off to keep Allied ships from being seen by the German subs. The U-boats landed eight people on Long Island, New York, and on the Florida coast. These Germans, who were to engage in spying and sabotage, were caught and executed.

As the Japanese captured Manila in the Philippines, American troops headed for Northern Ireland. These would be the first American troops to land in Europe during the war. About this time a Japanese sub fired shells at an oil refinery near Santa Barbara, California. June 3–6 was the turning point in the war in the Pacific when the American navy won the battle of Midway. It was during this battle the Japanese lost four aircraft carriers. The Americans lost the *Yorktown*.

U. S. Marines landed at Guadalcanal on August 7, while others landed in Morocco and Algeria in North Africa. From this point forward, the Axis powers would be on the defensive.

Despite conditions in other parts of the world, folks at home in Blackville and Healing Springs had good jobs, money to spend, and time for fun. The local movie theater showed *Casablanca, Mrs. Miniver,* and *Bambi,* and the radio broadcast popular songs: "Praise the Lord and Pass the Ammunition," "Don't Get Around Much Anymore," and "Jingle Jangle Jingle."

On February 2, 1943, the Germans at Stalingrad surrendered, and in July Allied forces invaded Italy. In the Pacific, the Americans had won the battle of Guadalcanal and the naval battles of Midway and the Bismarck Sea. This was good news. Everyone knew then the Allies would win the war, but no one knew how long it would take.

World War II was a period of extensive letter writing and there was a steady stream of letters and boxes to loved ones in service. Newspapers were read thoroughly and every radio news report listened to with care to learn what was happening where fathers, brothers, or sons were stationed. There was constant fear a telegram would arrive from the government announcing the death of a loved one.

Despite the improved job situation there were shortages of food and clothing. Shoe rationing began on February 2, 1943, which allowed only three pairs of leather shoes annually per person. Local farmers laughed about this since they were lucky to get one pair of shoes annually. In March, coupon books were issued for purchasing food. Sugar, meats, lard, and cheese were rationed.

The war did not end race riots. In Detroit, Michigan, whites protesting the employment of blacks clashed with blacks. Before the U. S. Army could stop the riot, 34 people were killed. That same year, a race riot in Harlem, New York City, resulted in 5 deaths and 410 injured.

To take their minds off the war for a while, folks in Blackville went to see movies—*The Song of Bernadette* and *Madame Curie*—and sang songs—"Mairzy Dotes," "Besame Mucho," "Do Nothin' Till You Hear From Me," "Comin' in on a Wing and a Prayer," and "They're Either Too

Young or Too Old."

World events progressed rapidly when the Allies landed in Normandy, France, June 6, 1944. This day is still known as D-Day. A few months later Paris was recaptured. In the Pacific, the Americans invaded the Philippines. Although the Germans released their secret weapon, the buzz bomb, on England, the war was coming to a close.

It was at this time that Lucian (Lute) P. Boylston, son of George W. Boylston, grandson of Austin Boylston, great grandson of George Boylston, and owner of Healing Springs, decided the springs needed eternal protection. After years of contemplation and discussion with friends, Lute decided to return the springs to their rightful owner for all posterity. He did this by deeding the property where the springs are located to "Almighty God."

State of South Carolina
County of Barnwell

KNOW ALL MEN BY THESE PRESENCE, That I, L. P. Boylston, believing myself of sound mind, and knowing the uncertainty of this mortal life, and remembering the gifts of Almighty God to me during my long life of over seventy six years, feel that I should return forever a part of which He, my god, has allowed me to possess and enjoy according to the laws of my country for many years, and feel that I should return to

Him the most treasured piece of this earth that I have ever owned and possessed, viz: one piece, parcel or lot of land measuring approximately one acre, with one of my Healing Springs or Flowing Wells situate thereon.

NOW. THEREFORE, for and consideration of my love and affection for my God, as herein above expressed, I do grant, release and convey to Him eternally the following:

All that piece, parcel or tract of land, situated, lying and being in the above State and County, measuring and containing approximately one acre, with one of my Healing Springs or Flowing Wells situated there on. The northern boundary thereof measuring one hundred and forty (140) feet and bounded by lands of my own; the eastern boundary measuring three hundred and fifteen (315) feet and ajoined by lands of my own; the southern boundary measuring one hundred and forty (140) feet and bounded by lands of my own, and the western boundary measuring three hundred and fifteen (315) feet and bounded by lands of my own.

TO HAVE AND TO HOLD all and singular the said before mentioned unto the said Almighty God forever; in Trust, nevertheless, for the public use, especially for the diseased or afflicted to use the precious healing water that flows from this God given source, reserving, however to myself, so long as I may live, full and complete control and supervision of the said described property herein conveyed.

AND I hereby constitute and appoint as Trustees to function upon my demise and to carry into effect the purposes of this conveyance, my only children, Virginia and Louise, and President of Furman University and his successors in office, and, in event of a vacancy in the office of either of the Trustees hereinabove named, the surviving two are empowered to select a third to fill such vacancy, and, in event of the failure on their part to so do, I empower and request Judge of Probate of Barnwell County to fill such vacancy, or to fill all vacancies when it may become necessary, and the said Trustees are empowered and directed to supervise and repair, if need be, the casing or piping of said springs so as to insure a continuous flow of the precious healing qualities of the waters of the Springs; It being historically true that the Indians who once possessed the land and waters realized and regarded it as Healing Gift to them from the Great Spirit, but I do not believe the white people, who dispossessed the Indians, ever appreciated the value of God's gift sufficiently to help in anyway preserve for posterity this gift of Almighty God to mankind, for several

white people have tried to destroy said Well
or efficacy of its waters during the time I
have owned it.

WITNESS my Hand and seal this 21st
day of July in the year of our Lord one thousand nine hundred and forty-four and in the
one hundred and sixty eighth year of the
sovereignty and independence of the United
States of America.

SIGNED, Sealed and Delivered
in the presence of,

L. P. Boylston

M. B. Whittle Jr. (witness)
B. F. Gardner (witness)

CONCLUSION

World War II came to an end and the service men and women came home. Each town and community celebrated their return. After a period of readjustment, many of the veterans decided to go to college under the G. I. Bill. Thousands of young men and women, who would never have been able to get a college education, were now off to continue their education. Most, once they received their college degrees, did not return to the farms or their hometowns. Thus, communities like Healing Springs and small towns like Blackville stopped growing. This trend continued across America. Many communities were saved when significant events, like the building of the Savannah River Site near Aiken, occurred.

Thanks to Lute Boylston, the Healing Springs will continue to flow and be available to everyone for generations. The next time you travel near Blackville, take time to stop by and drink the cool, healing water. By doing so, you will become a part of history.

SOURCES

BOOKS

Allen, Hervey and Carl Carmer, eds. *Rivers of America*. 1951.

Andrist, Ralph K., ed., and Edmund Stillman. *The American Heritage History of the 20's & 30's*. New York: American Heritage Pub., 1970.

Barck, Oscar Theodore, Jr., and Hugh Talmage Lefler. *Colonial America*. New York: Macmillan, 1958.

Barnwell County Heritage Book Committee. *Barnwell County Heritage*. Barnwell, SC: Barnwell County Heritage Book Committee, 1994.

Bass, Robert D. *Swamp Fox*. Orangeburg, SC: Sandlapper Publishing, 1954.

Beyer, Fred. *North Carolina—The Years Before Man: A Geologic History*. Durham, NC: Carolina Academic Press, 1991.

Boyer, Paul. *The Enduring Vision, A History of the American People*. Lexington, MA: D.C. Heath, 1996.

Boylston, Raymond P. *The Battle of Aiken*. Aiken, SC: Aiken Historical Society, 1964.

————. *Butler's Brigade: That Fighting Civil War Cavalry Brigade from South Carolina*. Raleigh, NC: Jarrett Press Publications, 2001.

————. *Edisto Rebels at Charleston*. Raleigh, NC: Boylston Enterprises, 2004.

———— and Samuel Boylston. *Boylston Family History*. Self-published, 1995.

Brown, Virginia Pounds and Laurella Owens. *The World of the Southern Indians*. Birmingham: Beechwood Books, 1983.

Cardwell, Donald. *The Norton History of Technology*. New York: W.W. Norton, 1995.

Cooper, Jacquelyn Williams. *Springfield, South Carolina: A Small Town Saga in Orangeburg County*. Springfield, SC: J.W.Cooper, 1988.

Culler, Daniel Marchant. *Orangeburgh District 1768–1868: History and Records*. Spartanburg, SC: Reprint Co., 1994.

Davidson, James West. *Nation of Nations: A Concise Narrative of the American Republic*. Boston: McGraw-Hill, 1999.

Devereaux, Margaret Green. *The Land and the People*. Columbia, SC: South Caroliniana Library.

Edgar, Walter. *Partisans and Redcoats: The Southern Conflict that Turned the Tide of the American Revolution*. New York: Harper Collins, 2003.

———. *South Carolina, A History*. Columbia, SC: USC Press, 1998.

Fleming, Thomas. *Liberty! The American Revolution*. New York: Viking, 1997.

Holmes, John W., ed. *Memoirs of Tarleton Brown, A Captain in the Revolutionary Army, written by Himself*. Barnwell, SC: The People Press, 1894.

Jennings, Peter and Todd Brewster. *The Century*. New York: Doubleday, 1998.

Lambert, David and the Diagram Group. *The Field Guide to Early Man*. New York: Facts on File, 1987.

Lorence, James J. *Enduring Voices*. Lexington, MA: D.C. Heath, 1993.

Maddox, Annette Milliken. *The Long Shadow of the Big Brick, A History of the First Baptist Church, Blackville, South Carolina, 1846–1996*. Blackville, SC: First Baptist Church, 1996.

McDonald, Everette Stanley. *The Story of Blackville, SC*. Blackville, SC: Blackville Area Historical Society, 1993.

———. *Natural History Buried in Blackville, SC Including Healing Springs and Slaughter Field*. Blackville, SC: Blackville Area Historical Society, 1993.

McGill, Ralph. *The South and the Southerner*. Boston: Little Brown, 1963.

Mills, Robert. *Mill's Atlas of South Carolina, 1825*, Barnwell District Map, surveyed by Thomas Anderson, 1818. Orangeburg, SC: Sandlapper Publishing.

Milling, Chapman J. *Red Carolinians*. Columbia, SC: USC Press, 1940.

Neuffer, Claude H. *Names in South Carolina*. Spartanburg, SC: Reprint Co., 1976.

Nies, Judith. *Native American History: A Chronology of the Vast Achievements of a Culture and Their Links to World Events*. New York: Ballantine, 1996.

Osborne, Anne Riggs. *The South Carolina Story*. Orangeburg, SC: Sandlapper Publishing, 1988.

Pursell, Carroll W., Jr., ed. *Technology in America: A History of Individuals and Ideas*. Cambridge, MA: MIT Press, 1981.

Reader, John. *The Rise of Life: The First 3–5 Billion Years*. New York: Knopf, 1986.

Reynolds, Emily Bellinger and Joan Reynolds Faunt, eds. *The County Offices and Officers of Barnwell County, S.C., 1775–1975: A Record*. Spartanburg, SC: Reprint Co. for USC Southern Studies, 1976.

Ripley, Warren. *Battleground, South Carolina in the Revolution*. Charleston, SC: *Post-Courier*, 1983.

Salley, A. S. *The History of Orangeburg County, South Carolina, from its First Settlement to the Close of the Revolutionary War*. Baltimore: Regional Pub Co., 1969.

Schlesinger, Arthur M. *The Almanac of American History*. New York: Putnam, 1983.

Trager, James. *The People's Chronology: A Year-by-Year Record of Human Events from Prehistory to the Present*. New York: Holt, Rinehart & Winston, 1979.

NEWSPAPERS, PERIODICALS, MAGAZINES

Helsley, Alexia Jones. "Historical Rivers of the Carolinas." *Carolina Living.com*. November 1, 2002.

Hughes, Bill. "Edisto, Chicora Indians." *The State* (Columbia, SC). October 18, 19__9.

King, Shannon. "Blackville Home to Mysterious Artesian Well." *The State* (Columbia, SC). July 3, 2000.

Quattlebaum, Myrtle. "The Waters are Healing." Blackville, SC: Blackville Area Historical Society.

"Religious Farmer Willed Healing Spring to God." *The Columbia (SC) Record.* June 1, 1978.

Roberts, Lori D. "They were the first South Carolinians. American Indians tell their own stories in resource book for teachers." *The State* (Columbia, SC). February 3, 2000.

South Carolina Wildlife Magazine. May–June 2000.

INTERVIEWS, PERSONAL CORRESPONDENCE, PRIVATE PAPERS

Barnwell County South Carolina Company B, South Carolina Artillery, South Carolina Volunteers, Confederate States of America, Papers. Barnwell County (South Carolina) Public Library.

Boylston Family Papers. Hemrick Salley Collection. Salley, South Carolina.

Healing Springs Baptist Church Records. Provided by Rev. David Grubbs.

McDonald, Stanley. Interview by author. Blackville, South Carolina. August 27, 2002.

O'Bannon, Joyce S., ed. *Barnwell's Tarlton Brown: Patriarch of a Civilization, Documents Related, and Revolutionary Memoirs.* Unpublished manuscript, Barnwell County (South Carolina) Public Library, 1970.

———. *The Story of Healing Springs Slaughter Field and The Natural History Buried in Blackville, South Carolina.* Unpublished manuscript, Barnwell County (South Carolina) Public Library.

Quattlebaum, Myrtle. Interviews by author. Blackville, South Carolina. August 27, 2002, and August 14, 2003.

Ross, Dan I. Interview by author. Blackville, South Carolina. August 27, 2002.

Sassaman, K.E., M.J. Brooks, G.T. Hanson, and D.G. Anderson. "Native American Prehistory of the Middle Savannah River Valley." Savannah River Archaeological Research Papers. South

Carolina Institute of Archaeology and Anthropology, University of South Carolina, 1990

LIBRARIES, HISTORICAL SOCIETIES, ORGANIZATIONS
Aiken-Barnwell Genealogical Society, Aiken, South Carolina.
Allendale Paleo-Indian Expedition, Institute of Archaeology and Anthropology, University of South Carolina.
Barnwell County Library, Barnwell, South Carolina.
Blackville Area Historical Society, Blackville, South Carolina.
Internet: Indian People of the Edisto River, Four Holes Indian Organization, Edisto Tribal Council, Inc.
Orangeburg County Historical Society, Orangeburg, South Carolina.

OTHER
Healing Springs Baptist Church, 1772–1972. Program for 200th Anniversary, October 8, 1972.
Post Route Maps of North Carolina and South Carolina 1896.
South Carolina 1820 Census.
South Carolina Tax Returns, Winton County, 1787–1800.
Topographical Map of North and South Carolina by J. H. Colton, 1861.
Winton (Barnwell) County, SC Minutes of County Court and Will Book, 1785–1791

ABOUT THE AUTHOR

Raymond Powell Boylston, Jr., is a South Carolina native, born January 28, 1930, in Aiken. Most of his early life was spent with his grandparents, Samuel and Olive Boylston of Springfield, South Carolina. Ray Boylston descended from the Boylstons and Reeds who settled in the Healing Springs area, along the South Edisto River just north of Blackville, in the late 1700s. While living in Springfield, Ray Boylston often visited Healing Springs and Blackville and drank from the cool springs.

In 1995, Boylston and his brother Sam, of Columbia, South Carolina, wrote the "Boylston Family History," which was the source of much information for this book. Ray Boylston is also the author of *Butler's Brigade* published in 2001, which describes the Confederate Cavalry Brigade in which his great-great uncles from Healing Springs served during the Civil War. He published in 2004 *Edisto Rebels at Charleston*, a book about two other great-great-uncles from Healing Springs who served in the Confederate Artillery on James Island near Charleston and in North Carolina.

Boylston graduated from the University of South Carolina in 1951, then served in the Army Chemical Corps during the Korean War. He was employed by the DuPont Company for twenty-two years in South Carolina, Delaware, and North Carolina. In 1973 he became Director of the Occupational Safety and Health Administration for North Carolina. Leaving OSHA in 1977, he served about two years as Safety Director for the American Textile Manufacturer's Institute. Thereafter, until his retirement in 1994, he served as vice president and president of ELB and Associates, Inc., of Chapel Hill, a safety and health consulting firm. During that period, he was an instructor at the University of North Carolina at Chapel Hill.

Boylston served on the Aiken County Historical Commission and authored a booklet on "The Battle of Aiken." An inscription by him about the battle is engraved on the battle monument in Aiken. He served as president of the American Society of Safety Engineers and is a fellow in that organization. Boylston is a member of the North Carolina Writers Network and the Raleigh Civil War Roundtable. He lives with his wife Bobbie in Raleigh, North Carolina. They have three children, seven grandchildren, and three great-grandchildren.

Barnwell Baptist Association,
192
Barnwell County Heritage, 7, 77
Barnwell State Park, 233
Barnwell, town of, 5, 81, 164,
173–74, 176, 178, 180, 185,
199
Barr, Henry, 148
Barton, Captain, 71
"Basin Street Blues," 232
Bates, James Arthur, 80
Battery Wagner, 162, 164
Baxley, John, 112
Beasley, Percy, 224
"Beat Me Daddy, Eight to the
Bar," 245
Beauford Bridge, 163
Beaufort District, 68
Beaufort, town of, 150
Beauregard, P. G. T., 146, 160–
61
Beech Island, 71
Belgium, 246
Bell, Cynthia Jowers, 132, 174
Bell, James, 132
Bell, John, 174
"Beloved Woman," 19
Ben John, 68
Bennett, Elizabeth. *See* Boylston,
Elizabeth Bennett
Bergen, Edgar, 242
Berlin, Irvin, 243
"Besame Mucho," 251
Best Friend, 130
Best, Clio Legard Bignon, 186
Best, Henry, 70
Best, Richard, 186
Big Band music, 231, 239
Bignon, Clio Legard. *See* Best,
Clio Legard Bignon
"Bill Bailey, Won't You Please
Come Home," 210

Bill of Rights, 105
Bismarck Sea, battle of, 251
Black, John Alexander, 128,
130–31
Blackville, town of, 1, 5, 7, 50,
56, 129–39, 142–43, 145–52,
154, 160–61, 171–75, 177–78,
180, 182, 188–92, 195–96,
199, 200, 202, 204–09, 211–
13, 215–26, 229, 231, 235–37,
239, 240, 244, 246, 249–51,
256
Blackville-Alston-Newberry
Railroad, 206
Blatt, Jake, 236
Blatt, Nathan, 236
Blatt, Solomon, 236
Blatt's, 236
"Bless 'em All," 245
"Bloody Bill." *See* Cunningham,
William
Bloom, E., 137
Bloom, family of, 112
Bloom, Pinckney, 137
"Blues in the Night," 249
Boiling Springs, town of, 71, 81
Bonaparte, Napoleon, 120
Bonnie and Clyde, 233
"Boogie Woogie Bugle Boy," 249
Bourguoin, Major, 68
Box, Mahulda. *See* Boylston,
Mahulda Box
Boy Scouts, 235
Boylston Landing, 1, 82, 121,
212
Boylston, Alice Hardin Cloud,
78–79, 81, 83, 94, 96–99, 123,
143
Boylston, Anne. *See* Staley, Anne
Boylston
Boylston, Annie, 94, 97
Boylston, Austin, 58, 94, 112,

265

Boylston, Susanna. *See* Adams,
  Susanna Boylston
Boylston, Thomas, 81
Boylston, Virginia, 254
Boylston, William (son of
  George and Alice), 94
Boylston, William (son of
  Thomas and Elizabeth), 81
Boylston, William Bennett, 78–
  79, 81–84, 96–98, 100, 105
Boylston, Zabdiel, 97
Brabow, Dr., 163
Branchville, town of, 173–74
Brannon, General, 156
Breeden, Gladys, 237
Brier's Creek, 55, 69
Briggs, Dr., 237
Brodie, Emma Porter, 179
"Brother Can You Spare a
  Dime," 231
Brown Cotton Gin Company,
  195
Brown, Barney, 128
Brown, Bartlet, 56, 70
Brown, John, 141, 145
Brown, Joseph J., 148
Brown, Mike, 200
Brown, Simon, 133, 204, 236
Brown, Tarlton, 55, 67–71, 73
Brown, Virginia Pounds, 22
Bryant, William, 67
Buck Rogers, 232
Buford, Abraham, 72–73
Buford's Bridge, 133, 187
Buist, Dr., 237
Buist, H. L., 236
Buist, J. L., 236
Buist, Sam, 236
Bull, General, 67
Bull, William, 119
Burnside, General, 162
Burton's Ferry, 55

Bush River, 44
Butler, A. P., 185
Butler, Eloise, 185
Butler, James, Jr., 75
Butler, M. C., 166, 185, 197–98,
  208
Butler, Pinkney, 148
Butler, William, 70
Butler's Brigade, 166, 170–71,
  186
buzz bomb, 252
"By the Light of the Silvery
  Moon," 218

C

Cabaniss, Alice, 77
Cadet Rangers, 167
Cain, family of, 58
Calhoun, John C., 41, 125
California, 135, 137
  Santa Barbara, 250
Camden, town of, 66
  battle at, 67, 72–73, 78
Camp Butler, 147–48
camp meetings, 120–21
Canada, 122
Cane Creek, 38
Cannon Bridge, 175
Caribbean, 116
Carolina Bays, 7
"Carolina Moon," 223
Carolina Railroad, 139
Carroll, Charles, 236
Carroll family, 80, 133
Carroll, Julia, 113
Carroll, William B., 147–48
"Carry Me Back to Old
  Virginny", 206
Cartwright, Edmund, 114
Casablanca, 250
Cassidy, Hopalong, 238
Castle Pinckney, 188

267

Boylston, Mary Crum Moorer
Morgan, Daniel, 78
Morgan, John H., 156–57
Morgantown, 156, 180
Morris, Darling P., 148
Morris, family of, 58
Morris, R. B., 230
Morris Ford, 68
Morris Island, battles on, 162,
164–65, 185
Morrison's, 236
Moses, Franklin F., Jr., 195
Moslems, 114
Mott, Captain, 68
Mount Carmel, 72
Mrs. Miniver, 250
Mulberry Grove Plantation, 115
Mumford, John, 68
Murrow, Edward R., 242
Mutiny on the Bounty, 239

N

National Archives, Washington,
DC, 84
National Association for the
Advancement of Colored
People (NAACP), 215
National Geographic, 12
National Grange, 202
National Industrial Recovery Act
(NIRA), 227
National Recovery Administra-
tion (NRA), 227
Netherlands, 88, 246
Nevada, 135
Nevils, Cynthia, 137
Nevils, family of, 161
Nevils, Jessie, 137
Nevils, Lewis, 137-38
Nevils, Martha, 137–38
Nevils, Mary, 137
Nevils, R. Frank, 148, 164

"New Deal," 227
New England, 34, 53, 88–89,
122, 134, 202, 209
New Jersey,
Hoboken, 127
New London, town of, 35
New Mexico, 135
Clovis, 12
New York, 128
Long Island, 250
New York City, 80
Harlem, 251
News and Courier, 202
Ninety Six, town of, 66, 72, 76
Nix, Robert, 148
North Augusta, town of, 16, 18,
20, 197
North Carolina, 38, 41, 52–53,
60, 67, 78–79, 122, 171, 182,
187, 205, 229
Asheville, 229
Aversboro, battle of, 181
Bennett Place, 181, 185
Bentonville, battle at, 181, 185
Charlotte, 38
Durham, 181, 185
Fayetteville, 181
Goldsboro, 181
Greensboro, 78, 181–82, 185
Guilford Courthouse, battle
of, 67, 78
Kinston, battle at, 171, 185
Kitty Hawk, 212
Outer Banks, 149
Salisbury, 79
Wilmington, 78, 185
Northwest Ordinance of 1787,
105
Northwest Territory, 105
Norway, 246

White Cliffs of Dover," 248–
49
"There's a Long, Long Trail,"
218
"They're Either Too Young or
Too Old," 251–52
3rd South Carolina Cavalry
Regiment, Company D, 187
3rd Virginia Regiment of Conti-
nentals, 72
This is London, 242
Thomas, family of, 112
Thomas, Lowell, 226
Thomas, Rhubin, 112
Thompson, Colonel, 68
Thornton, Mary. See Boylston,
Mary Thornton
"Three Little Fishes," 243
Three Musketeers, The, 238
Tilden, Samuel J., 201
Tillman, Benjamin R., 207–08,
211
Titanic, 215
tobacco, 19, 205
Tobin, Cornelius, 129
Toby Creek, 50
Tolbert, James, 190
Tom Mix westerns, 222
Topper site, 11–12
Trail of the Lonesome Pine, 239
Treaty of Paris, 84
Treovithick, Richard, 127
Trexler, H. Flowe, *v*
Turkey Creek, 50
Turner, Captain, 75
Turner's, 236
Twain, Mark, 201
typhoid fever, 173, 246

U
Uncle Tom's Cabin, 138
United Daughters of the Con-

federacy, 166
United States Constitution, 85,
105
University of South Carolina
Institute of Archaeology and
Anthropology, 12
Utah, 135

V
Valentino, Rudolph, 222
Van Buren, Martin, 131
Vasquez de Ayllon, Lucas, 28, 31
Victoria, 106
Victoria, Queen of England, 210
Vikings, 12
Vince, Joseph, 69-70
Virginia, 38, 41, 45, 52–53, 60,
67, 70, 78, 81, 166–67, 171,
173, 180–82, 185–87, 205
Albemarle County, 56
Appomattox, 187
Atkinson's Farm, battle at, 170
Big Bethel, battle at, 149
Brandy Station, battle of, 166–
67
Cactus Hill, 11
Chancellorsville, battle at, 162
Charles City Court House,
battle at, 170
Charles Station, battle at, 170
Charlottesville, 171
Cold Harbor, battle at, 185
Drewry's Bluff, battle at, 170
First Manassas, battle of, 185
Five Forks, battle at, 171
Fredericksburg, 162
Gordonsville, battle at, 170
Harper's Ferry, battle at, 141
Haw's Shop, battle of, 170
Jackson Hospital (Richmond),
171
Manassas, battle of, 149